Praise for *Redirecting*

D1372536

"Susan Vitalis opens her heart to share her faith journey to inspire all of us to chase our dreams and to live an authentic life of significance. Vitalis uses her personal experiences to guide you to find your passion, embrace your gifts, get involved, and take the lead in your own life. *Redirecting: Discovering Hope in the Unexpected* will encourage, motivate, and challenge you to live the life you were meant to live, and in the process, leave your mark on this world."

—**Kerstin Kealy,** news anchor and producer,
WDAY Television

"Dr. Vitalis tells a riveting story of faith and vocation that all of us can learn from. Her life mission is filled with promise and despair . . . faith challenges and victories. Susan provokes all of us to stand back and look at our own lives and be grateful our jobs can also be an amazing calling and faith-filled journey."

—**Kevin Wallevand,** television news reporter, WDAY,
two-time Emmy and Edward R. Murrow Award winner

"In the midst of an incredible career, unexpected hurdles threatened to derail both passion and personal identity, leaving Susan confused and searching for God and His ultimate plan for her life. In *Redirecting: Discovering Hope in the Unexpected,* you will be inspired and encouraged by Susan's humor, heart, and faith as she shares her unique and remarkable journey. It is a must read!"

—**Judy Siegle,** two-time Paralympian, author,
Living Without Limits

"This book is for those who are looking for something without knowing what they are searching for, for those who know what they are seeking but do not know where to find it, and for those who simply need a spark to ignite the fire that burns deep inside. *Redirecting: Discovering Hope in the Unexpected* is full of passion, faith, and heart, serving as a rallying cry to inspire us to reach out our hands and our hearts to touch the lives of those across oceans and in our own backyards. With warmth, humor, and honesty, Dr. Susan Vitalis recounts how God's calling on her life has changed over time, from medical missions in Africa, to motivating young adults to live out their passions in the world. In times when we are often overwhelmed with stories of violence and despair from around the globe, this book shines out as a light in the darkness, illustrating love, joy, and a fierce determination to live 'a life of significance.'"

—**Emily Ronsberg,** '19, biology and premed student,
Concordia College, Moorhead, Minnesota

"An exciting, authentic read with a story so compelling that you will hold your breath waiting for the next episode. You will be led to look inward at your vocation and outward at your present state. *Redirecting: Discovering Hope in the Unexpected* will relate to your call, vocation, and thinking outside the box at whatever age you are. You will laugh and cry. The author's lived experiences and spiritual journey will inspire and motivate you to seek God in all things."

—**Barbara R. Holm,** spiritual director, retreat leader,
writer, counselor

"In *Redirecting: Discovering Hope in the Unexpected,* Dr. Susan Vitalis offers an open and refreshing look into the self-doubt that is so prevalent within us (yet rarely revealed) as we approach our vocation. Within Dr. Vitalis' inspirational stories lie an underlying comfort with personal limitations, knowing that in weakness we are made strong. I invite all Christians considering a first career, undergoing a life transition, suffering from anxiety, or simply seeking to discern each day's call to join her in being similarly vulnerable. Although our egos are tantalized by the extraordinary, more often the 'still, small voice' is calling us to worship as we live out the ordinary. As Dr. Vitalis' career expectations were thwarted by a serious knee injury, an ensuing complex neurological pain syndrome, and a traumatic brain injury, she responded to the call to love others in day-to-day acts of listening and caring. God speaks to us through her experience: 'Ad lib and add love.'"

—**Roger Lindholm, M.D., FAAFP**

"*Redirecting: Discovering Hope in the Unexpected* is a compelling look at the work we do, and how it morphs into a vocation, a passion, a calling."
—Alyson Green, MLIS Librarian

"If you are searching for significance and wondering, 'Why am I here and what am I to do?' *Redirecting: Discovering Hope in the Unexpected* will resonate with you. It will bless anyone who reads it and encourage you as you seek to understand life more."
—Robyn C. Moore R.N., MSN, CPNP, Least of These Ministry, World Gospel Mission, Kenya

"If you are at a point in your life where you need God to 'split the Red Sea' for you; if you are discouraged and feel attacked on all sides, read *Redirecting: Discovering Hope in the Unexpected*. Listen to this testimony, and behold the God of the Bible, who is alive today and who loves to take care of His kids."
—Shane Barnard, vocals, guitar, songwriter, Shane and Shane

"What an experience to have been able to read the thought-provoking message of the power of God's amazing grace in the pages of Dr. Susan Vitalis' book, *Redirecting: Discovering Hope in the Unexpected.* Dr. Vitalis has experienced life in many different situations, but throughout some of the most difficult or subtle changes, we are able to feel her understanding of God's call to life as God touches her through many very special people and situations. As I began reading, the feelings of strength and love compelled me to continue. I would recommend this book for anyone, whether their life is a massive struggle or a cozy, warm world. God's love abounds in everyone's needs. Thank you, Susan, for sharing God with us."
—Rev. John G. Krueger, pastor, ELCA (retired)

"When Dr. Susan Vitalis was my high school math student and basketball captain, I became convinced she would do something remarkable with her life; however, remarkable doesn't begin to describe her life of service. In her book, *Redirecting: Discovering Hope in the Unexpected,* Dr. Vitalis addresses the challenges of trying to listen to God's voice calling us to serve, when so many other voices bombard and distract us. Dr. Vitalis has spent her entire life listening to the small, quiet voice of Jesus whispering in her ear, 'Truly I tell you, just as you did it to one of the least of these who are members of my family, you did it to me.' (Matthew 25:40). Her passion for helping those in need has been and will continue to be recognized by anyone who meets her. Her message for each of us in *Redirecting: Discovering Hope in the Unexpected* is to keep our hearts, minds, and ears open so that we can discover our own true calling. This is a challenge that should ring true for all people of faith."

—**Marc Langseth,** math teacher and women's basketball coach (retired)

"Dr. Susan Vitalis beautifully captures the triumphs, tragedy, and grit of medical missions in the developing world. Be drawn in by her master storytelling ability in *Redirecting: Discovering Hope in the Unexpected*. An excellent read for college students searching for mission and purpose, and churchgoers looking to transition from lethargy to action."

—**Hannah Rhinehart,** team member, Mission Medics to Nicaragua

"Experiences in life do not happen by accident. Even before the universe was created, God had us in mind, and He planned us for His purposes. The powerful stories shared in this book help us to understand why we are alive and God's amazing plan for us—both here, now, and into eternity. Susan's insights may help you to transform your answer to life's most important question: What on earth am I here for? A book of challenge and hope, I believe *Redirecting: Discovering Hope in the Unexpected* will be treasured by generations to come."

—**John Parkes, Jr.,** Chief People Officer & co-owner, Murdoch's Ranch & Home Supply, Montana

"This is a rich, arresting story of faith active in love. If one is looking for religious sentimentality, this is not the book. If one is looking for flesh and blood religious realism, this is the book. In addition, Vitalis writes with ease and clarity. Dr. Vitalis writes with the authenticity of a practitioner, the credibility of one who 'walks the talk,' and the passion of one who is called to ministry. *Redirecting: Discovering Hope in the Unexpected* is filled with arresting stories that illustrate the nexus of faith and life. Fundamental questions of faith are examined in the context of medical practice, and, occasionally, personal angst. Susan's exposition on vocation is especially useful to seekers of every culture and generation. The reader will be inspired and enlightened on these and other fundamental issues."

—**Paul J. Dovre,** President Emeritus, Concordia College

"'A beautiful testimony of faith, brought me to tears, and couldn't put it down,' best describe *Redirecting: Discovering Hope in the Unexpected* by Dr. Susan Vitalis. This is for anyone who struggles with life's questions or who ponders the meaning of life. Loved it!"

—**Mary Duquet,** avid book reader

"How do we listen for God's voice in our lives? What if we don't particularly like what we hear? In *Redirecting: Discovering Hope in the Unexpected,* Dr. Susan Vitalis gives us a very personal and inspirational account of a journey that begins in Minnesota and ultimately leads to some of the most dangerous places in the world. This is what it means to listen for God's voice, and then follow God's direction—regardless of the consequences. What we see is a life of true vocation, unwavering love, and ultimate trust."

—**Dr. Mark Jensen,** Professor, Concordia College

"Susan Vitalis' devotion, passion, and spiritual enlightenment shine through in her life and on every page of *Redirecting: Discovering Hope in the Unexpected.* A wonderful read for book clubs, confirmation classes, Bible studies, and anyone who has a stirring in their heart for service to others, or just wants a great book to read. This book reads like a friendship that endures; one full of thought-provoking conversations, laughter, tears, and stories of adventures that won't let you put the book down."

—**Anne Goldsmith,** health educator, Melrose Center, St. Louis Park, Minnesota

"*Redirecting: Discovering Hope in the Unexpected* is what finding and walking out God's will looks like in a well-worn pair of hiking boots. It's about how we all can find, then step into the adventure that awaits us if we are willing to leave our comfort zones of faith behind—so that we can see the lives of true significance and lasting legacy that our Creator has created us all for."

—**Michael W. Franklin,** Christian bookseller, Jesus follower

"Dr. Susan Vitalis is a healer, a compassionate visionary, and a woman of vibrant faith. Her book *Redirecting: Discovering Hope in the Unexpected* is a compelling read, filled with stories of life's challenges, tragedies, hopes, and dreams. *Redirecting: Discovering Hope in the Unexpected* is the memorable journey of a marvelous young woman doctor as she ministers her way through the lives of some of God's most unforgettable people. Stories of pain-filled struggles, hope, and triumph will enthrall and challenge the reader. You will walk with Susan as she journeys through a world in which she faithfully and humbly encounters the active and loving presence of our God. Dr. Vitalis becomes, as we are all called to be, the very hands and heart and face of our caring God as we see God's vivid encounters with so many of our special brothers and sisters. Her book *Redirecting: Discovering Hope in the Unexpected* will encourage each reader to boldly and faithfully continue on their own journey and to open their very lives to the living and transforming presence of God's love and calling."

—**Rev. Ernest (Ernie) A. Mancini,** Lutheran pastor,
college pastor, college administrator

"Reading *Redirecting: Discovering Hope in the Unexpected* has made me a better person—reading this book will do the same for you."

—**Laura Locher,** devoted friend

"*Redirecting: Discovering Hope in the Unexpected* is an adventuresome read for anyone discerning a meaningful life of service. Dr. Susan Vitalis' work deals with challenges, courage, and commitment. Here is a study in personal possibilities if one heeds the relentless call of God to serve by being sent forth in this world of need. *Redirecting: Discovering Hope in the Unexpected* is an uncommon story of victory over adversity...service over self...and joy in surrender. It is a must read for anyone searching for meaning and a life truly dependent on God's abundant grace. Vitalis' legacy to her readers is one of desire to walk with anyone who wanders in the wilderness of doubt and to bring faith and fulfillment to life."

—**Kathryn Benson,** RN, Concordia College Health
Center Administrator

"EVERYONE should read this book! Dr. Susan Vitalis gives me confidence, and this book inspires me to just be me by following my heart and by taking chances."

—Taya Rostad, nine-year-old book lover

"Dr. Susan Vitalis courageously unveils her personal journey to existential and spiritual clarity in *Redirecting: Discovering Hope in the Unexpected*. This tale by a Lutheran girl from Fargo who becomes a Johns Hopkins-trained physician and medical missionary, only to suffer a series of almost unbelievable travails, will capture the hearts of every reader. While framed in her own sphere of experience, the simple messages resonate as truths for all people, regardless of culture, religion, or origin of suffering."

—Lucinda Bateman, M.D., Medical Director, Bateman
Horne Center of Excellence, Salt Lake City, Utah

"In *Redirecting: Discovering Hope in the Unexpected*, Dr. Susan Vitalis communicates from her heart and leaves behind any form of deception or pretense that almost always impedes communication and hinders getting the job done. If you are worn out with the 'church goers' with their petty piety, and would like to get an insight into how Jesus would truly wish to see life, then *Redirecting: Discovering Hope in the Unexpected* is a must read."

—Jay Olson, pharmacist

"Dr. Susan Vitalis gives us a candid behind-the-scenes view of being involved in short-term medical ministry in her new book, *Redirecting: Discovering Hope in the Unexpected*. My missions journey coincided with Susan's at Tenwek Hospital, and I can definitely relate to many of her African adventures. If you've ever grappled with physical and spiritual challenges, you will be encouraged by Susan's journey. If you've struggled to discern God's voice in the midst of a busy and loud world, if you are looking for fulfillment beyond imagination, or if you're wondering whether God is speaking to you about using your medical skills, really any skills, in cross-cultural ministry, this book is for you."

—Joy Phillips, career missionary

"Susan's stories unveil a fascinating life of risk and adventure, but more significant is her witness to how God called her to a career in medical mission in spite of her feelings of inadequacy. She vulnerably shares her journey through other lands, health issues, and mission, offering inspiration for anyone who doubts that God can use them."

—**Rev. Doug and Monica Cox,** Executive Director of
Global Health Ministries

"Too many people trudge through their lives and careers, in a rut, refusing to challenge themselves largely because they don't believe in themselves. In her book, *Redirecting: Discovering Hope in the Unexpected,* Dr. Susan Vitalis helps us see that our potential and possibilities are limitless if we choose to follow our God-directed passions. The path might not be easy, but Vitalis, who has faced her own challenges, shows anyone doubting their destiny, that to underestimate yourself is to underestimate God. A good read for those looking for inspired direction."

—**Tracy Briggs,** columnist, video host, and Honor
Flight Coordinator, WDAY Honor Flight

"At a time when some Third World countries needed medical assistance, Dr. Susan Vitalis felt the need to help. In her book, *Redirecting: Discovering Hope in the Unexpected* she relates what happens when a person says yes to the GREAT COMMISSION, not heeding the risks. Dr. Vitalis shares her life story with passion and adventure, making the connections of how God prepared, guided, and led her to Somalia, Sudan, Rwanda, and beyond. This book inspires and affirms one's mission in a world of need."

—**Pastor Johan and Sonja Hinderlie,** former
Executive Director and Program Director at Mount
Carmel Ministries

"In *Redirecting: Discovering Hope in the Unexpected,* Dr. Susan Vitalis invites us on a captivating journey through her extraordinary life. Vitalis shines through her words, describing life moments with humble sincerity and humor to teach us all how to live a life of significance. Reading this book feels like a conversation with a good friend or mentor, and we cannot help but be encouraged, inspired, and changed for the better even after just a few pages. Through her words and example, we understand that we are meant for more than the ordinary. We find true joy in discovering our purpose in this life, and we learn to thrive."

—**Nan Kennelly, M.S., CCC,** owner/speech-language
pathologist, Onword Therapy

"I have known Susan Vitalis over the span of two decades. We have been to the uttermost parts of the world together, serving children and families in villages few ever knew existed. She has and continues to let no personal adversity quench her passion and desire to share God's love and message of hope to a physically and spiritually hurting world. She speaks with wisdom and experience, which has been borne in the crucible of suffering. Her faith and her resilience have been tested and she continues to stand on the foundation of faith in Jesus Christ. She is giving us the privilege of seeing the road God ordained for her. In *Redirecting: Discovering Hope in the Unexpected,* there is much we can learn from her journey and insights."

—**Kirk A. Milhoan, M.D., Ph.D., FAAP, FACC,**
Medical Director, For Hearts and Souls

REDIRECTING

Discovering Hope in the Unexpected

Susan M. Vitalis, M.D.
Foreword by David Stevens, M.D., M.A.

Redirecting
Discovering Hope in the Unexpected
By Susan M. Vitalis, M.D. © 2018

Lead Editor: Anna McHargue
Cover Direction: Marina Alcoser
Interior and Cover Design: Fusion Creative Works, fusioncw.com
Photography: Susan Vitalis

Print ISBN: 978-0-9997602-0-8
eBook ISBN: 978-0-9997602-1-5

Book production by Aloha Publishing
All biblical references are from NRSV

For more information, visit SusanVitalis.com.

Published by Be Still and Know

Printed in the United States of America

To My Family:

*Thank you for the love, support, and encourage-
ment you have given me throughout the years,
on the roller coaster ride of my life. Words cannot
express the depth of my love for you.*

Contents

Foreword

Susan Vitalis is one of the most extraordinary physicians I know, and I know an extraordinary number of physicians as the CEO of the Christian Medical & Dental Associations, the largest professional organization of its kind in the world. I first met Susan when she came to help at Tenwek Hospital in Kenya for three months in 1990, where I served as the hospital's CEO. Her work ethic, medical expertise, compassion, and love for the local people made her stand out among the countless short-term physicians who traveled overseas to help. We became good friends, a friendship that has lasted for more than 25 years.

I can smell the scents and feel the heat she describes, and I know the people who fill her stories in her captivating book. I led the effort she was part of to relieve the suffering of people in Mogadishu, where more people were dying due to the lack of basic healthcare than were starving from a fearsome famine or being murdered in the street-to-street fighting of their civil war.

REDIRECTING

I led the relief team that landed on a makeshift dirt airstrip and traveled upriver to Ulang, Sudan, in a boat so heavily loaded with our small team, tents, and supplies that we had two inches of freeboard between us and a crocodile-infested river. Susan loved others and served them with joy, despite being in the most difficult living conditions you can imagine, in the midst of an Ebola-like epidemic of relapsing fever with a 50 percent mortality rate. It was a disease easily cured with a few cheap tetracycline tablets, but they had none, so there were 400 fresh graves at the edge of the village, dug the month before we arrived.

I was in charge of the team she served on in Rwanda during the genocide of 1993. To open the largest hospital in the capital, our team had to remove the dead bodies of the patients who had been slaughtered in their beds and then stare down the killing teams that tried to enter the hospital to kill the patients they had admitted for treatment.

Like Susan, I've seen the worst of evil and the best of good people who tackled it head on. I've seen despair turn to hope. I've seen faith and faithfulness that dwarfs my own amidst ceaseless suffering and too-frequent death.

Susan is more than an extraordinary physician. She is an extraordinary woman and gifted author. Despite her many accomplishments, she is permeated with humility. She considers herself simply an ordinary servant of an extraordinary God who trusts Him enough to follow His command to love her neighbors as herself. Her neighbors don't live next door but in foreign and forgotten corners of the world where people live an ignored existence of desperation and despair.

Her book is a gift to you. She has traveled tens of thousands of miles, sacrificed hundreds of thousands of dollars of income, put her life at risk in war and epidemic zones, and given up her comfort to learn the priceless principles she is freely sharing with you. As she states in the first chapter of her book, the goal of this book is "to prepare you for living a life of significance."

Think about it. Your life will one day be over. What are you spending it on? Are you selling your life for too little, or instead pursuing big, scary, audacious goals? God has given you talents and passions, but if you only look at those, you will still aim too low until you realize He also gives you His strength, His guidance, and so much more. The key to unlocking your true potential is to seek His will, grasp His calling, and exercise your faith by trusting Him.

Go out on the proverbial limb, and then hand God the saw to cut it off so you are only dependent on Him. That is what Susan did, and God used her to change the world in ways she never imagined.

I was captivated by this book. I could hardly put it down. With engaging humor, inspiring stories, and captivating honesty, *Redirecting: Discovering Hope in the Unexpected* shows you the way to true fulfillment and joy.

Susan went down the road less traveled and is eager to show you the way. Relish your journey. You will be delighted you took the trip!

David Stevens, M.D., M.A.

REDIRECTING

When the runners came from Bethlehem
All breathless with good news
They were passing a baton forward through time
The commission, from God's lips to our ears
Carried by His saints two thousand years
Connects us all to the same lifeline
As I fix my eyes ahead
I can feel the Spirit's breath . . .

And I can hear the mission bell ringing out loud and clear
It's the revolution Jesus started, and it's here
Echoing across the world from the shores of Galilee
I can hear the mission bell call for you and me
I wanna run with fire
It's my heart's desire
Lifting Your love higher

In the history of our faith's arrivals
Great awakenings, Welsh revivals
Saints and martyrs, summoned by a new birth
Patrick's save of the Irish nation
William Carey's expectation
Lambs & lions
Called to the ends of the earth
Gotta put my hand to the plow
Not looking back, not now . . .

—Newsboys, *The Mission*

Introduction

Not many people have the opportunity to publish an en-
hanced version of their book within a year of their first launch
day. For a variety of reasons, I am in a position to do just that!
Redirecting: Discovering Hope in the Unexpected is a revised
version of *Still Listening: How to Hear God's Direction at Life's
Crossroads*. All of the content from *Still Listening* is also in
Redirecting. In addition, there is more content, many more
pictures, and questions to ponder alone or in a group setting.

Years ago, when I first started writing while actually thinking
about creating a book, I was focused on my memories and
experiences in Africa . . . in Kenya, seeing hundreds of people
die from meningitis due to lack of vaccine and antibiotics;
in Somalia, watching the faces of the women and children
we were helping turn from gratitude to distrust after a U.S.
Military Black Hawk helicopter was shot down in the streets
of Mogadishu by militants and civilians; in Southern Sudan,
being evacuated under gunfire while leaving the Sudanese
behind; and in Rwanda, suffocated by the oppression and

evil because of the bloody massacres of the genocide. Of course, there were wonderful experiences working in Africa as well. I love Africa, and part of me will always be in Africa. Even though I have blonde hair and blue eyes, and am mostly of Scandinavian heritage with a touch of Irish, I'm sure if I had my DNA analyzed I would find a tiny drop of African blood in me. It would only be fair since I have literally left a lot of my blood with the Africans. The spirit of Africa will always be in my marrow.

When I tried to write a book about my African experiences, I found that it was becoming more like a travel log, which could be interesting; however, that wasn't my goal in writing. Instead, I want my book to be something that will encourage, motivate, and change the reader in a positive way.

There are very good reasons why I am writing this book at this point in time. The foremost reason is because God is clearly calling me to do it now. Throughout my life I have tried, at least for the most part, to follow where God is leading and do as Jesus would do.

Sometimes, He makes His path clear and sometimes, not so much. When it comes to writing this book at this time, God has been bending over backwards to compel me to recognize the opportunity I have before me. No more dilly-dallying. No more excuses. He has laid out the path and I am starting my trek, inviting you to join me.

Another reason I am writing is because a lot has happened in my life over the past few decades that has given me better insight into life, and how to deal with pain, change, loss, and abuse of power, for a start. Now I have a message that is clear.

INTRODUCTION

I have been blessed beyond words but I have also suffered and been lost, wandering in the wilderness too many times with so many questions and no obvious answers.

This book was written to inspire and educate, to prepare you for living a life of significance. If I can help you find your spark and then have it ignited, I will be blessed. I want to share what I have learned throughout my life to make it easier for those of you who already embrace your passion, yet don't know what to do with it; to inspire you who are holding back because you think what you want to do is too big or you aren't qualified or think someone else can do it better. And for those of you who are wandering in the wilderness? It is my hope that my reflections can help you find your way out.

It is also time for me to pass the torch. It's time for a passionate new generation to go out into the world to help those in need. Living out the life God created for us is crucial to living a life of significance. For me, helping those most in need is a fire in me that burns from my skin to my bone marrow, from the top of my head to the bottom of my feet, ignited from my heart. That's how God created me. It is not a decision I made, rather a voice I heard and a passion I embraced. Because of limitations, I can no longer go to places I have gone before, even though I see there is still so much work to be done. With this work, I am passing the torch, hoping to find people with a spark that is ready to be ignited.

Finding our calling and uniqueness is crucial to finding true joy. Many of us are satisfied living in the status quo, finding our groove that eventually becomes a rut and we don't realize there may be more to living, more out there for us to do. When was the last time you were excited to get out of bed in the morning? If you can't remember, chances are you have not experienced a passion that is unique to you for a very long time, if ever. Sometimes normalcy in life can be a respite after a time of chaos, and we can embrace those times as needed rest. The apathy I'm talking about is when we are passive, day after day, waiting for something better to drop at our feet; days that turn into months and then years, where the only spark in our life is our pilot light that is enough to keep us going, but that needs a spark to ignite us to follow the flame to a new level of joy. With this book, you may see that it's time to find your passion so that you might live a life of significance, regardless of your circumstances. I have spent many of my days pursuing what I saw as achievements, rather than looking at what I was being called to do. Finding my passion started with discovering who I am and who God created me to be. My prayer for you is that I can save you years of struggling by helping you start down your path of finding your passion and significance, knowing there will be pain along the journey, changes that drop us to our knees, and situations that hit us on our blind side.

All of us are unique. I know that sounds obvious. We all have our own gifts and flaws. No one has exactly what you have to offer. When I was at Christikon Bible Camp in Montana the summer after 7th grade, we were studying 1 Corinthians. In Chapter 12, verses 14-21, the writer Paul talks about the importance of every part of the body; such as, if we were all made feet, how could we see? My counselor compared it to a Big Mac, which may sound silly, but it stuck with me. At that time the McDonald's jingle was, "Two all-beef patties, special sauce, lettuce, cheese, pickles, onions on a sesame seed bun." The all-beef patties may think they are the most important part of the sandwich, but without the pickles it would not be a Big Mac. God created me, and you, in a specific way for a specific time and specific purposes. I'm just fine being a sesame seed. You can be the special sauce.

This is not to say that God can only use us in one way and if we stray from His path we're in big trouble. Not so. His first desire is that we have a close relationship with Him. He sent His son Jesus into the world—the Word made flesh, Immanuel—to forgive our sins, save us from ourselves, and show us how to love. Truly love. The more we live in God's presence, the more we can understand what He has in store for us, taking one step at a time. He is present everywhere, and He invites us to step into His arms where He will keep us safe in the center of His will.

When I say safe, I don't mean that God will keep us from getting hurt or even dying. But we will be exactly where He created us to be. In Romans 8:35-39, Paul says, "Who will separate us from the love of Christ? Will hardship, or distress, or persecution, or famine, or nakedness, or peril, or sword? As it is written, 'For your sake we are being killed all day long; we are accounted as sheep to be slaughtered.' No, in all these things we are more than conquerors through Him who loved us. For I am convinced that neither death, nor life, nor angels, nor rulers, nor things present, nor things to come, nor powers, nor height, nor depth, nor anything else in all creation, will be able to separate us from the love of God in Christ Jesus our Lord." This describes so well what it means to be safe in the center of God's will.

Death has stared me in the face many times, and somehow I seem to come out the other side still alive in this world. To say I was never anxious or even a bit afraid in these circumstances would mean I was not being honest with myself. However, I do know that when I am in situations where I am consciously aware that I can live or die; knowing that I am where God wants me to be gives me comfort. As David says in Psalm 56:11, "In God I trust; I am not afraid. What can a mere mortal do to me?"

Before I go on, I need you to know that I am not a trained pastor and have no earthly credentials to teach others what the Bible says or means to say. My dad, sister, and brother-in-law are pastors and will attest to the fact that I contact them frequently with questions about what the Bible is saying about this or that. The Bible sums up my faith best in Ephesians 2:8-10, "For by grace you have been saved through faith, and this is not your own doing; it is the gift of God—not the result of works, so that no one may boast. For we are what He has made us, created in Christ Jesus for good works, which God prepared beforehand to be our way of life."

In my own words, my faith has evolved from what I was taught as a child, what I questioned as an adolescent, and what I experienced through life, which has brought it to what it is today. Basically, I am a Lutheran by heritage and worship in a Lutheran church, but it does not define my faith. Rather it is a lens through which I come to understand God. I am a Christian because Jesus has claimed me as His own. I believe the Bible to be true, and I know Jesus came to earth and died on a cross to save me from my sins. He desires a personal relationship with me, and calls me to live my life as an example of His with the big implication of that being to love everyone. Deep breath. There it is in a nutshell. My intent is not to preach, but rather to share my story. I believe there may be something for people of all faiths to glean from this book and in my story you may discover a bit of your own story.

Recently, I was asked to ponder the following two questions: "What does it mean to pass the torch?" and "What do I want my legacy to be?" My response to both was immediate and with authority, surprising me with the speed and clarity. To the first question about passing the torch I said, "I want to educate the younger generation, to motivate and encourage them to get involved in the world in a positive way, using my life experiences as a guide." To the second question about my legacy I said, "I want to be remembered as someone who lived a life reflecting Christ—nonjudgmentally helping the least of these."

Uff da, I still have a lot to learn!

REDIRECTING

Sometimes I think
What will people say of me
When I'm only just a memory
When I'm home where my soul belongs

Was I love
When no one else would show up
Was I Jesus to the least of us
Was my worship more than just a song

I wanna live like that
And give it all I have
So that everything I say and do
Points to You

If love is who I am
Then this is where I'll stand
Recklessly abandoned
Never holding back
I wanna live like that

—Sidewalk Prophets, *Live Like That*

CONCEPT 1

Go Deeper to Discover Your True Potential

*We know we were made for so much more
Than ordinary lives*

*It's time for us to more than just survive
We were made to thrive*

—Casting Crowns, *Thrive*

If you would have asked me during my first year of college if I would ever be a doctor, I would have laughed and snorted, "No way! I'm going to be a high school math teacher." My first calculus class quickly changed my sights from becoming a math teacher to a biology teacher. I was good at math, but quickly found that I enjoyed biology much more.

Why did I laugh at the thought of becoming a doctor? I am a great minimizer. During the summer between my second and third year of college at Concordia College in Moorhead, Minnesota, I worked with a friend who was pre-med. By this time I was questioning my desire to be a teacher, and my favorite classes were Anatomy/Physiology, Biochemistry, Genetics, and Biomedical Ethics. Hmm . . . I started to see a pattern there. My friend asked me why I wasn't interested in becoming a doctor and I responded, "I'm not smart enough." Now it was her turn to laugh and snort, "What are you talking about? You're as smart as all the pre-meds!" Huh. Maybe I could get into medical school.

Deciding to go to the homecoming football game my fourth year of college ended up being one of the most pivotal days of my life. Ann, the friend I was sitting with at the game, asked me where I was applying for medical school to which I responded, "I'm hoping to get into the University of North Dakota." Fargo was my home-town at the time. She casually said, "You ought to apply to Johns Hopkins." My turn again to laugh and snort, "Are you kidding me? There's no way I could get into the best medical school in the country!" She was serious. "My uncle graduated from Concordia and then went to Johns Hopkins. He liked it so much that he stayed as a Pediatric Orthopedic Surgeon. I'll have him send you an application." Fine. I changed the subject, figuring she wouldn't follow through.

Two days later I received a package from Dr. Vernon Tolo with an application and letter that said something like, "Ann told me you're interested in applying to Johns Hopkins Medical School. My family and I love it here. I sent the application by overnight mail because the deadline is soon. I hope to see you in Baltimore next year!" Oh my goodness. Now I was in a conundrum. He went to all the time and expense to get me the application, so how could I not apply?

And yet, it cost $50 to apply and the questions were in-depth and personal, which would take time. But Dr. Tolo and Ann went to so much trouble, I couldn't let them down. So, in my mind, I spent a lot of time on an application that would get me nowhere and wasted $50. Once again, I was minimizing and underestimating myself.

When I received the acceptance letter to Johns Hopkins School of Medicine, part of me was excited, but a bigger part was terrified because I knew they must have made a mistake. It's the only thing that made sense to me. Ultimately, I decided to accept the offer, and resolved to spend every waking minute for the next four years studying medicine. On the first day of orientation, when there was a short pause between speakers, one of my fellow classmates said, "Do you know what they call the person who graduates last in their med school class? M.D." That broke the ice for all 120 of us as we realized we were all terrified to some degree. As we looked around, we were surrounded by the people who would help each of us get through the next four years, on the path to becoming lifetime friends.

Underestimating our ability is, in reality, the same as underestimating God's ability. Philippians 4:13: "I can do all things through Him who strengthens me." And we know what God can do. Absolutely anything and everything, more than our minds can even grasp. And we have God's power within us.

John 15:7 says, "If you abide in Me, and My words abide in you, ask for whatever you wish, and it will be done for you." So if we underestimate what we can do, we are underestimating what God can do.

REDIRECTING

The same power that rose Jesus from the grave
The same power that commands the dead to wake
Lives in us, lives in us

The same power that moves mountains when He speaks
The same power that can calm a raging sea
Lives in us, lives in us
He lives in us, lives in us

—Jeremy Camp, *Same Power*

So how do we tap into God's power? We have access to it all as long as we have faith to receive it. Sometimes it takes something dramatic to bring us to our knees and ask for power and strength because when things are going well, we take the credit and forget that it's really not us in control.

There was another defining moment in my life when I underestimated myself. But this time I came to realize that by doing so I was underestimating God at a time I needed Him in all His glory and with all His power. Let me set the stage for you: I was in Kenya on my first mission trip right after finishing my Family Medicine Residency program. It was the longest day of my 29 years on earth.

The day started in the usual way: Dr. Roger Lindholm and I made the uphill walk to Tenwek Hospital in rural Kenya, from our "home away from home." Roger and his family are dear friends from Minnesota who slaved through residency with me. While in Kenya, I lived with Roger, his wife, Joan, and their two young daughters, Leah and Jamie. Roger and I arrived for doctors' report at 8 a.m., short of breath from the exertion. My body never fully adjusted to the altitude of 6,800 feet, and my lungs could never seem to find enough oxygen in the thin air, particularly on this day since I had been in the country for less than a week. Morning report was a time for all the doctors to meet and hear what had transpired during the previous night from the on-call physician. After the report, we prayed together and then spread out to our respective wards, where we were quickly swallowed up and immersed in work.

Around 8:30 a.m., after seeing only a handful of patients on my ward, there was an overhead page for any doctor to go to the outpatient department STAT. At least that's what it sounded like. The hospital was made up of several buildings, but they did not all have speakers, so people would shout loudly into the audio system to make sure they were heard by all. A combination of poor quality equipment that created more static than distinguishable words, plus a frantic Kenyan trying to speak English but in panic, often reverting to the local Kipsigis language, made it difficult to understand the pages. But I thought I caught the words "doctor" and "STAT," and this was confirmed when my Kenyan nurse pushed me out of my ward and pointed to the outpatient department.

I ran there with Wendy, a nurse from the United States, close behind. When we arrived we saw a man who appeared to be in his early 20s collapsed on the floor. Since we were the first to arrive, we started CPR; soon Roger also arrived and jumped into action. Initially we didn't have an interpreter, but someone wheeled in a crash cart for us. To say that we bumbled through the code is an understatement. I don't think the crash cart had been updated for a decade or two, a conclusion I came to quickly with one glance at the cart. There was no defibrillator, and the equipment that was there was ancient and rusted. At least we could figure out most of the medicines since the names were, for the most part, recognizable. We worked on this patient for about an hour, but could not revive him. All we knew about him was that he had walked into the out-patient department, unaccompanied, and collapsed. I have no idea what led to his death.

As we were cleaning up the mess we had made during the code, there was another page: "Dr. Susan Vitalis to Ward 118, STAT!" Ward 118 was my women's ward, so I sprinted down to find the nurses doing CPR on a 16-year-old patient with asthma and congestive heart failure (CHF). In the United States, when we hear that someone has CHF, we picture an elderly person. But in Kenya and other African countries, that is not always the case. This patient had congestive heart failure that could be traced back to an episode of strep throat that went untreated. The streptococcal infection traveled from her throat to her blood, causing rheumatic fever, and then the infection seeded on her heart valves, causing rheumatic heart disease that eventually led to CHF. Her asthma led to respiratory arrest, and her heart was having difficulty keeping up with the increased need for oxygenated blood throughout her system. We tried to resuscitate her for about an hour, but were unable to revive her.

As I was explaining to her parents what had happened, I was overcome with the feeling of defeat. How could I convey to them, through a translator, why their 16-year-old daughter had died? I took a chance by taking their hands in mine; not knowing if this was culturally acceptable. After all, I had only been in their country for a few days. But they squeezed my hands and held on tight, so I figured it was the right decision.

I knew that if the girl would have had access to the medical care we provide in the U.S., she would not have died from asthma and CHF. For one, the strep infection would have been treated either at the point when she had strep throat or rheumatic fever. And her asthma could have been managed with inhalers and other medicines if treatment had been started earlier. Occasionally we had inhalers available that were brought in by doctors coming from the States, but there were never enough for the large demand. At that point in time, we had eight inhalers in the pharmacy, and that was only because I had brought six with me. I don't remember what I told her parents, but I vividly remember the feeling of inadequacy.

Just as we attempted to start rounds again, Roger's voice came over the loudspeaker: "Code in Ward 3," Roger's female ward. Once again, I found myself sprinting across the hospital grounds to another crisis. As soon as I arrived, Roger sent me looking for a mask and breathing bag since his patient was unable to breathe on her own. Both fortunately and unfortunately, I knew right where they were, since I had just used them on my ward. I darted back to Ward 118, grabbed the equipment I needed, and ran back to Ward 3. Thankfully, adrenaline allows our bodies to do more than we could under normal circumstances. I would normally be jogging, but adrenaline kept me sprinting. I found myself thinking of my hurdling days in high school track because I was jumping over wheelchairs and beds, some unoccupied and some piled with people, all of whom were wearing a universal startled look on their face. The distance was never more than 100 yards, but the obstacle course made it feel longer.

When I returned, Roger filled me in on this patient. She was a 38-year-old pregnant woman with nine children, who had come to the hospital that morning with a nine-day history of headache. She was completely alert and communicative when she first arrived, but subsequently stopped breathing while her heart kept beating.

We intubated her in order to provide her lungs with the most oxygen possible while we hoped and prayed she would come around. Her heart was beating fine, so if we could just get her breathing again on her own, we could start looking for a cause for her headache. We knew we couldn't stay and bag her all day, but we kept at it for about an hour. By then her pupils were fixed and dilated, which suggests irreversible brain damage, and she was not showing any signs of breathing on her own. So we quit breathing for her and then waited for her heart to stop beating from lack of oxygen; this took about ten minutes.

Our guess was that the patient had an abscess, tumor, or something else in her head that caused swelling, which gave her headaches.

In the States, we could have put her on a respirator and then obtained a CT scan to see what was going on in her brain. But we weren't in the States. I was starting to learn that the only way to survive working in a country without the same resources available as in the U.S. was to separate myself and see them as two separate countries instead of trying to make comparisons. This was a tough lesson that didn't totally sink in until subsequent trips to various African countries.

By about 4:30 p.m., I had seen all the patients in my wards. I headed to the outpatient clinic to see if they needed my help, hoping they would not so I could catch my breath. Unfortunately, the patients were terribly backed up and they desperately needed me.

Are you kidding me? When will I have time to breathe? I somehow managed to swallow these questions before they came out of my mouth.

The clinic was entirely a walk-in clinic, so there were no appointments. We had no control over how many patients were seen in one day. The first patient I saw in the clinic was a 15-year-old girl who had come to the clinic because she had been raped twice by the same man. Understandably, she was an emotional wreck. (So was I, for that matter.) Once again, it was very difficult to talk through a translator about highly emotional, sensitive issues. As I was talking with her, I heard a brief moment of static on the loudspeakers and knew, even before the words came out, that there was another crisis somewhere. "Any doctor to Labor and Delivery, STAT!" I thought to myself, "Please, not Labor and Delivery."

For the fourth time that day, I found myself sprinting across the hospital grounds, not knowing what I would find. I soon came upon a midwife delivering a baby that was in the breech position (feet first instead of the normal head first presentation). She had the baby's body out of the birth canal, but the head was stuck. Another doctor arrived at the same time as I did, so we each took a side; he pulled on the baby from below, and I pushed on the abdomen from above. We weren't making much progress, and the baby was getting bluer and floppier. We tried pulling her out with forceps with no success. The other doctor said, "The baby is not going to survive. It's time to use the destructive instruments to get this baby out."

I didn't know what these instruments were specifically, and I wasn't ready to find out. After all, this baby still had a heartbeat. We compromised by giving it another minute before getting out the despised instruments. I went back to pushing on her abdomen with renewed energy; I did not want to destroy this baby. Finally, with all of us drenched in sweat and breathing as though we had just finished a marathon, the head popped out! Hallelujah! But our work wasn't finished. The baby had a weak heartbeat and wasn't breathing on her own. So, for the fourth time that day, we started resuscitative efforts.

I thought, "No problem. Babies are born with weak heartbeats all the time. And many need help breathing initially. She'll come around." To my great disappointment, she didn't. My feelings of inadequacy continued to mount. She was a full-term baby who was healthy in every way except that her head didn't fit through the birth canal.

This was the fifth death of the day, counting the three-month-old fetus that died with her mother who, at the age of 38, was the oldest person to die so far that day. It was 6 p.m., and I knew I had to return to the outpatient clinic to finish talking with the rape victim and continue to whittle away at the people left waiting.

As I was walking to the outpatient clinic, I was overcome with a sense of inadequacy, powerlessness, and weariness. I questioned how I could survive the next three months. I pictured myself decimated, piece by piece, left in the middle of Africa to die. Okay, this may sound a little melodramatic; however, at the time, not so much. It was then that I realized my belief had to dig deeper than it ever had before, or I would be crushed—especially since I was on call that night, which meant my day was actually just beginning.

I was in over my head. There was no way I could keep going. I started to question if I was cut out for mission work after all. God had been preparing me for this moment for years. And then it hit me. It was God who directed me to Tenwek Hospital. Not me. I was looking at my situation through my limited brain with my limited resources, again underestimating what I could do. But God has no limits and, through Him, I can do anything. I knew I couldn't survive on my own without turning everything over to God. What a relief!

I believe that day was the first time I came to the realization that I could no longer underestimate myself if God was with me.

And the thing is, God is always with us, whether we feel His presence or not. There is absolutely nowhere we can go to escape Him. So if God is available to me at all times, and He has no limits whatsoever and if I have the faith to know this to be true, I have no limits. Wow! What a concept! Maybe it was time to quit underestimating myself. Joshua 1:9 popped into my mind, "I hereby command you: Be strong and courageous; do not be frightened or dismayed, for the Lord your

God is with you wherever you go." I then knew my survival depended on turning everything over to the Lord, daily letting go of myself, and becoming one with Him.

At that point, I was certain that I was safe in the center of God's will. I still might die, but I was assured of His Presence every step of the way. My faith went from being two feet wide and one inch deep to becoming a bit narrower and a tad deeper.

Just because God has the ability and power to do everything doesn't mean He will do what we want or think He ought to do. He has the big picture in sight when we see only a tiny drop of water that is soon absorbed by the ocean. Not that long ago, the consensus was that the world was flat. One could not see beyond the ocean, therefore nothing existed past where the ocean dropped into an endless abyss where adventurous sailors fell to their demise, an assumption made when they did not return home. We now know the earth is round—and so much more.

There was a specific day that I realized I had learned something from my previously described longest day. I was awakened in the middle of the night while on call and summoned to the procedure room with no explanation of what to expect. When I walked into the room, the patient was lying on the bed, smiling, and greeted me with, "Chamage" (cha-ma-gay), the local Kipsigis greeting, translated into English means, "Do you love yourself?" I replied, "Mising" (me-zing), translated "very much."

A nurse was at the head of the patient, cleaning what appeared to be a wound. The patient said he had been fighting with his neighbor and was hit on the top of his head with a panga, a long, curved machete blade. What happened next, I did not see coming. I looked over the nurse's shoulder at the wound and saw a deep laceration that went through his scalp and skull, which means I was looking directly at a small part of his brain trying to squeeze its way through the unexpected slit. *Call the neurosurgeon,* I thought instantly. *Wait a minute. I'm the doctor on call, which means I'm also the neurosurgeon on call. Uh?* I quickly thought back through my years of training and confirmed what I already knew to be true. I had never seen an injury like this before. In U.S. medical schools the motto is, "See one, do one, teach one." I was facing, "See one, and figure it out."

I went into my stitching mode, surprisingly calm, and got to work. First I cleansed and sterilized the wound as best I could, going way overboard with the cleaning solution. After all, this was his brain. Thankfully, the panga blade stopped before cutting into the brain. To be honest, medically it was quite fascinating. I gently tucked the brain back inside the skull and pulled the edges of the bones together as tightly as possible. I did not have the equipment needed to suture the bone but got as close as possible with the periosteum (the membrane covering the bone) and started putting in stitches. Many, many stitches. Once I was sure the skull was as secure as I could get it and the brain safely inside, I stitched the next layer until I finally pulled the skin together with my last layer. Unfortunately, there are not a lot of layers between the skull and skin. If his hair were longer, I would have tied that together as a final touch. It looked quite good, if I may say so myself. I gave him some antibiotics, admitted him to my men's ward, and went back to bed.

When I gave report the next morning at doctors' rounds, I realized I had stayed so calm because God's strength was in me, and with His help I had nothing to worry about. My treatment was better than no treatment at all. And I had no control of the outcome. I did my best and left the rest in God's hands. The fact that the man walked out of the hospital a few days later, seemingly as good as ever with maybe a lingering grudge against his neighbor, is nothing short of a miracle. God can do anything, but He needs us to be His vehicles to work through. I wish I could say that I stayed that confident all the time, every time, but that would not be the truth.

For a long time, I've worked on how to listen to God. But I continue to struggle. It would be so nice if God would write clear messages and display them behind small planes that fly over parades. Instead of a banner that says, "Shop at Everts Lumber and Hardware. Great sales!" the banner could read, "This is God speaking. Don't do it. Give the money to your neighbor in the yellow house two doors down who can't feed her children." Unfortunately, He doesn't work that way. We have to tune into His whispers and nudges and recognize them when they come. I sure wish I was better at this. It seems the only times I really try to listen to what God is telling me is when I have a big decision to make. What He really wants is for us to have a relationship so close to Him that we function in sync. Oh, my goodness, I am not there yet.

Dave, a friend of mine, relayed a time when he clearly heard God talking to him. This is a great example of how God may speak to us. He was serving on the staff of a prominent church when a denominational leader called him about a church that was looking for a senior pastor. He asked him if he would consider the position and consent to being interviewed by their board members. He and Kathy, his wife, were very content in their current situation and were not looking for a change. This time, though, the offer came out of the blue, so they decided to consent to the interview. Maybe God was calling them to a position where they were more needed.

There were no problems with the interview with the exception of the fact that about three-fourths of the way through, Dave sensed a change. As he says, "I've always been fairly adept at what I call 'discerning the room.' That is to say, knowing the direction the meeting is headed and picking up signals of what people might be thinking." As the interview was concluding, Dave knew the board was very pleased as questions turned toward logistics and timing of his call. The mood of the room was light, positive, and relaxed; with the exception of Dave's spirit. He was inwardly alarmed because while he sensed their openness and acceptance, he also sensed within his own spirit that this was not the situation for him. The church board was wondering when he could start, while Dave was wondering how he could gracefully leave the room.

The next day he was notified that the board unanimously voted to call him as their next pastor. Now the ball was in the hands of Dave and Kathy. While they continued to feel with fairly strong certainty and peace that they should stay where they were, those around them, from church leaders to close friends, felt the opposite. They were told he would be a fool not to take the position, that it was the right move for everyone, and word even got around that they had an exciting opportunity presented to them that they would probably be accepting. Everyone but God said, "Go." They could feel in their hearts that God was truly telling them, "Stay." They were certain that they should let this opportunity pass, while everyone else told them to grab it and run.

The opportunity never left Dave's mind and he started to wear down. One night while driving home from a meeting, exhausted from all the confusing thoughts and conflicting messages, in desperation, he finally asked himself, "Alright, what happens if I just say *yes*?" In his own words he explained what happened next: "Immediately, something forcefully rose up inside of me and shouted, 'No! That is NOT the right decision.' Was it me coming to my senses? Did I experience an awakening? Was it a moment of clarity? No. I don't know for sure, but I believe it was the Holy Spirit reminding me to follow what my heart knew was right. Because it's what He had put there."

Dave and his wife listened to God, followed their hearts, and were at peace when they turned down the position. A few months later, they discovered that circumstances had begun to develop in the church he turned down that would have been disastrous for Dave and his family. This was further confirmation to him that it is best to listen to God and your heart over everyone else.

In contrast, sometimes confirmation comes through other people. In early 1995, I flew to Kigali, Rwanda, to help get their hospital up and running after the horrendous genocide that occurred the previous year. While most of the massacres occurred in 1994, there were still killings during my time there. Even though the Tutsi tribe had declared victory over the Hutu tribe, the country was still in anarchy.

As soon as I stepped foot off the plane onto the runway in Kigali, I felt a pit in my stomach. Where did that come from? All I knew at the time was that I was very uncomfortable. Was it the bombed-out buildings, including the airport? No, I had seen much worse than that in Mogadishu, Somalia. Was it concern over my safety? No, I had been evacuated out of Southern Sudan under gunfire less than a year prior and didn't have this feeling. What was happening? This "feeling" was new to me. I continued through the airport, armed guards everywhere (just like Somalia), my luggage and I were thoroughly searched, and I hoped I would quickly see someone I knew. Finally, my ride arrived and it was Jen, a Canadian friend I had worked with in Somalia. Fantastic! Now I would surely feel better. The pit in my stomach became a little more bearable until we arrived at the house where we were staying. The pit became the Grand Canyon as I was given a tour of the house, being told how they had to remove several dead bodies and scrub down blood that was everywhere. Since the house was full, I stayed in a tent in the backyard with Karen, a nurse with whom I immediately became best friends.

However, to my dismay, the pit in my stomach turned to anxiety that eventually almost paralyzed me. I began to think that I had misread God and wasn't supposed to be in Rwanda. For the first time ever, I thought about money. Why am I spending so much money to be here while I could be making a lot of money if I just kept working in the States? Wow. Where did that come from? At the time, I didn't know what was going on, but after a few days I knew I had to get out of there. Paul and Jan, the leaders of the group and a couple I trusted and respected immensely, especially after spending time with them in a bomb shelter in Southern Sudan surrounded by gunfire, suggested I go to Nairobi, Kenya, for a few days to discern what God was calling me to do. I was ready to fly straight home; however, I knew they were right and I needed a safer and closer place to figure things out.

I stayed at a guesthouse run by the organization with which I worked. I spent the next several days reading the entire New Testament, praying, fasting, and even calling Johan Hinderlie and Marva Dawn, friends whom I had consulted in the past concerning spiritual matters. After about a week, I was feeling that I should return to Rwanda. Or shouldn't I? Doubts kept creeping in until I received confirmation in an unusual way. At least, it felt unusual at the time.

On Sunday evening, I started to feel anxious. When I went to bed, I could not sleep. I don't know how to describe what happened except I knew Satan was trying to take hold of my soul. It was the worst feeling I have ever experienced. And that says something after the dangers I had survived in the past. I put my headphones on and played Christian music. I prayed continuously, and I mean continuously, all night. When I couldn't think of words to say, I would recite the Lord's Prayer and would intermittently throw in something like, "Get away from me Satan, I have been washed by the blood of Christ, and you have no power over me." I could not wait for morning to come to get me out of this darkness. Monday was an exhausting day, and I learned that whatever

I was battling was big. I still didn't know what it was, but it was definitely much bigger than me.

The next day I went to a conference center outside of Nairobi where a missionary conference is held every two years. It was great to see people I had worked with at Tenwek Hospital, and they were surprised and happy that I came uninvited for the day. What happened next, I did not see coming.

Dora Wesche, the wife of a general surgeon at Tenwek and a prayer warrior, called out my name. I turned and gave her a big hug. She held onto my shoulders, looked directly into my eyes as she said, "Susan, I had no idea you were in Kenya. God awakened me Sunday night with you on my mind, and I was up all night praying for you!" I kept staring into her eyes as I was momentarily struck speechless. She broke the silence by saying, "What brings you to Africa?" Oh, my goodness, where do I start? I gave her a brief synopsis of what had happened since stepping foot off the airplane in Kigali. She said, "Satan is working hard to keep you out of Rwanda." There was my confirmation, coming from a woman I hadn't seen in years and wouldn't have seen if I had not chosen that day to go to the conference.

I returned to the guesthouse that night knowing exactly what I was supposed to do—and that meant I was just to *be*—to be a force of goodness and light. If Satan wanted me *out* of Rwanda so badly, God must surely want me *in* Rwanda. It was then that I realized this was a spiritual battle, pure and simple, and I was to return to Rwanda for the sole purpose of being a light in the darkness. What I had felt when I first arrived in Rwanda was the spiritual oppression and immense darkness that suffocated me, and I didn't recognize it. I didn't care what I would do in Kigali—I'd be willing to do absolutely anything, sweep floors and clean bathrooms—as long as I was a light in the darkness. Period. And, here, Satan's darkness went deep. But let me clarify: My idea of Satan is not a red man holding a pitchfork surrounded by flames. Rather, he is like a breeze that is felt but not seen. Madeleine L'Engle explains it well in her book *A Wrinkle in Time*. Her description of the character walking through darkness is spot on. She writes, "The coldness deepened and swirled all about her and through her, and was filled with a new and strange kind of darkness that was a completely tangible thing, a thing that wanted to eat and digest her like some enormous malignant beast of prey."[1] That is what I felt.

I had learned another lesson: When God puts someone in my mind, completely out of the blue, He means for me to act—to pray. It's what I know I am called to do. Am I perfect at this every time? Not even close. Instead, I am a work in progress who is trying to get it right.

We started the chapter talking about how we often underestimate ourselves and, by doing so, we also put limits on God who, in reality, is limitless. If I were to say that I no longer underestimate myself, that would not be true. The difference now, as opposed to my earlier years, is that I am quicker to recognize the conundrum I put myself in, and the box I put God in, when I don't recognize my full potential. My goal is to help Him do the work that needs to be done here and now. This will be a lifelong learning process.

Build Your kingdom here
Let the darkness fear
Show Your mighty hand
Heal our streets and land
Set Your church on fire
Win this nation back
Change the atmosphere
Build Your kingdom here
We pray

—Rend Collective, *Build Your Kingdom Here*

CONCEPT 2

Find Your True Calling

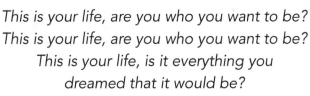

This is your life, are you who you want to be?
This is your life, are you who you want to be?
This is your life, is it everything you
dreamed that it would be?
When the world was younger
and you had everything to lose

—Switchfoot, *This Is Your Life*

Why is it that so many of us are interested in what job a person has? When we initially meet someone, our first question is usually, "What's your name?" which often is followed by, "What do you do? What is your job?" I didn't think much about this until I suddenly became unemployed. Whenever I hear the uncomfortable words, "So, Susan, what do you do?" I struggle with my response. I try to justify why I am unemployed by going into a long, confusing dialogue that leads to either more questions or the person saying, "That's nice," as they quickly move to the next person in the room. Likewise, talking about my vocation—my life's work—just adds to the confusion. "I currently don't have a job, but my vocation is pretty cool. I help people around the world in medical and nonmedical ways." Then they ask, "Are you a nurse?" "I wasn't tolerant enough to be a nurse, so I became a doctor." "So why is your vocation not your job?" "Typically, a job requires payment." "Why aren't you making money working as a doctor?" "It's a long story." As they walk away I can hear them mutter under their breath, "That's a weird one."

I'm not the only one in this predicament of not knowing how to answer the question about a job. Many people are laid off, between jobs, or on disability. Whatever the case may be, the question, "What do you do?" inevitably leads us to an unsatisfying answer. Indeed, the more we try to justify our answer, the more we dig ourselves into a hole. What would happen if everyone held up a united front and instead of answering the question, "What do you do?" with a job description, we said, "My vocation is medicine, helping those in need, and writing." For someone else it might be, "My vocation is making people laugh. I have a talent for helping people see the positive side of life rather than the negative. I also fix cars." Many of us think of our job and vocation as the same thing; however, that is not necessarily the case. According to Merriam-Webster, the definitions are quite different:

> **Job:** the work that a person does regularly in order to earn money: something that requires very great effort

> **Vocation:** a strong desire to spend your life doing a certain kind of work: the work that a person does or *should* be doing

Vocation can be looked at as a tripod where you need support from all three legs to keep from falling. One leg is what we *like* to do, our passion, deep desire, something that ignites our spark and fans our flame. Another leg is what we are *good* at doing. We may have a passion to play professional basketball, but don't have the ability to bounce a ball and run at the same time. The third leg is *filling a world need*. Our depraved world is waiting for people like us to tackle one small part of a humongous wound.

I can't say it any better than Frederick Buechner, "The place God calls you to is the place where your deep gladness and the world's deep hunger meet."[2] Stop reading for a moment, take a deep breath in and out, and now read the quote again. That's vocation in a nutshell. The needs of the world seem endless; however, we are called to use our gifts in a way that helps one of the world's many hungers. In order to accomplish this, we must be doing something that we are competent to do.

Vocation is a journey, a pilgrimage that we undertake where the road is not straight and roadblocks materialize when least expected. Some of us wait for our vocation to find us, waiting for that specific sign that will give us direction. There may not be a specific sign, but instead a strong momentum going in a particular direction. Move with it. This is an evolving process with more than one path that may change with our life experiences. We may not like every step of the process, but we are moving; sometimes forward, sometimes backward, sometimes sideways, and sometimes in a dizzying all-directions-at-once pace.

The key to finding our true vocation is to discover who God created us to be by considering our strengths and weaknesses, what makes us tick, what makes us cringe, and to take note of the sparks we feel in life so they can be ignited. A spark is felt at our core when we hear or experience something that resonates with us. Goosebumps (chicken skin) are also helpful.

In 2004, Concordia College Chemistry Professor Mark Jensen and I had a discussion about health vocations. He had been thinking about starting a health vocations class for first- and second-year students, and asked my opinion about whether or not it would be worthwhile. "Absolutely," I said. With further discussion, we discovered Mark and I were on the same page from the get-go. Through a "Call to Service" Lilly grant that was given to Concordia College, the first health vocations class was born in 2007. Today, each class session discusses a health care profession and is taught by someone in the community from that field. I cover the class on missions. For some, the class confirms what they already thought they wanted to do. For others, the class clarifies a path that was unclear. Universally, the students are challenged to look at their future in the context of vocation and spirituality rather than just finding a job.

Some people find their vocation as an extension of their job. Two friends have done this in an exceptional way. First is Kevin Wallevand, who works as a television news reporter for WDAY, a local news station in Fargo, North Dakota. His vocation, in his words, is to "tell the stories of those doing awesome things both home and away." What I see as the application of his calling is to help people by covering stories that are honest, issues that need to be addressed, acknowledging people who are doing great things, and always leaving the viewer wanting more.

Kevin majored in broadcast journalism. He said, "I fell into it." During his last year of college, he interned at WDAY and was hired as soon as he graduated. He liked the immediacy of the news and, as a reporter, found he was chasing whatever was breaking. It wasn't until he experimented with feature stories and documentaries that he realized his true vocation and passion were still evolving. Before this revelation, to him, he had a *job*.

Kevin has managed to work his vocation into his job. We still see him reporting current events on the evening news, but it has been through his documentaries that he has made his mark. Documentaries have allowed him to take time to develop a story that ultimately has motivated people to do something that can change a life—or several lives. That's vocation. That's passion. That's a calling. He has been to Peru, Vietnam, Angola, Haiti, Kosovo, the Middle East, and he accompanied me to Mongolia to cover the story of Munkhbayar and Batchimeg, who came to Fargo for heart surgery (the documentary is "Flight for Life"). His vocation has continued to develop and grow in Haiti, where he has been part of a medical mission 18 times and counting. His role has grown from being the one to document what others are doing to being an integral part of the planning, fundraising, and even assisting in surgery, among other medical needs. He has been nominated for several Emmys and has won three. In October 2016, he accepted his second Edward R. Murrow award in New York City for winning the best news documentary for his work on "Trafficked," which concerns sex trafficking in western North Dakota during the recent oil boom. His work changes people for the better.

Tracy Briggs is another person who has pursued her vocation. At the time of her vocation revelation, she was a morning radio host on 970 WDAY. One Sunday, while getting ready for church, she saw a story on a news program that literally brought her to tears. The topic was on Honor Air Flights, which flew WWII veterans to Washington, D.C., to see the WWII monument, among other sites. With tears and mascara running down her face, she told her husband, Mark, about this great story and his response was, "You should do it here." For the rest of the day, she was obsessed with the idea. She wrote a proposal and by the end of the next day, her plan had made its way up the ranks to the boss. Tracy was flabbergasted when it was approved that very day. She got home, laid on the floor, and thought, "What have I done? I'm not up to this." When her husband and daughters walked into the room, one look at Tracy led Mark to say, "So the boss didn't approve it? You're disappointed?" Tracy said, "No, it's a go and I'm terrified!"

The next year was a whirlwind for Tracy. She was working 12-hour days and raising two young daughters while attempting to accomplish something that had never been done in the Dakotas or Minnesota. She was determined to have an honor flight program in Fargo. With a great committee and wonderful community support, in May 2007, people from the extended North Dakota and Minnesota community watched the wheels of an Airbus 320 lift off the ground carrying 103 WWII veterans to Washington, D.C., to see the WWII monument for the first time. An additional 82 people were needed as escorts, support, and media, which exemplifies the enormity of the event.

This flight was one of the first Honor Flights in the nation, and the first in the Upper Midwest to send WWII veterans to see their memorial in our country's capital. By responding to her calling and passion that Sunday morning, Tracy started a ripple effect that keeps on going. Since 2007, there have been seven flights that have sent around 1,000 WWII and Korean vets to Washington, D.C., and the program has expanded to Bismarck, North Dakota, and Grand Forks, North Dakota, with 14 flights already in the books. Tracy hopes to expand the program to include Vietnam veterans. Wow! That's a calling!

Throughout my life, I have had a variety of jobs; however, my vocation, calling, and passion is medicine, which for me, means taking care of people—body, mind, and spirit. It fits the three legs of the vocation tripod. I like it, I'm good at it, and it fills a world need. Paraphrasing Frederick Buechner, quoted above, medicine is the place where my deep gladness and the world's deep hunger meet. I get goosebumps just reading that sentence. I realize my passion is something I must pursue, and through this book I hope to encourage you to do the same.

As I stated earlier, my initial plan after graduating from high school was to be a math teacher. My reasoning for that was because I was very good at math, and what else do you do with a math major except teach? Looking back, I realize that math wasn't my favorite subject—that honor goes to biology. One distinction in finding our vocation is to pursue what we most enjoy, not what we think we ought to do, or what we're the very best at doing, or what family, friends, and the world think we ought to do. We need to be true to ourselves and the gifts God has given us.

My senior year in high school, I received the science award for being the best student in the sciences. Mr. Alby, my physics teacher, approached me after the awards ceremony and asked, "Do you know what it means to receive this award?" I had no clue what was in his mind, but the first thing to come to mine was what I told him, "I guess I'll be taking a science class next year." He smiled and walked away. Little did I know how that conversation would change the course of my life.

During my first year of college, I did not enjoy calculus, but absolutely loved Biology 101—the class I felt I must enroll in because of the science award. It did not take me long to change my major from math to biology. Since I was already thinking I would be a teacher, I just switched my sights to becoming a biology teacher. What I had forgotten was being a teacher wasn't necessarily what I was interested in doing, but rather the only thing I could think of to do with a math degree.

In medical school, I continued to do what I most enjoyed. I loved every rotation and couldn't imagine giving up any of it, so it made sense to specialize in Family Medicine.

But I noticed something. During medical school, anytime there was discussion about work in Africa or other underserved areas, I felt a spark. I specifically remember driving from the University of Minnesota to my apartment in Hopkins after going to a required lecture on work that was being done with refugees from Thailand who lived in

Minneapolis and St. Paul. During the lecture, I felt the spark as never before. As I was driving west on I-394, passing under Hwy 100, the spark became a flame. I knew that I would be going to Africa. I didn't know when or for how long, but I was going.

After residency, I had the opportunity to work at Tenwek Hospital in Kenya for three months. Prior to leaving the U.S., I had a job waiting for me at Park Nicollet Urgent Care Clinic in Minneapolis, Minnesota. I chose urgent care because I loved the excitement of not knowing what I would face each day, and I also quickly learned that it gave me the flexibility I needed to do short-term mission work. I chose Park Nicollet because they were willing to give me that flexibility.

I headed to Kenya thinking that I would put in my three months, return to working urgent care in Minneapolis, and comfortably live happily ever after in the suburbs. That was not to be the case. My undeniably strong desire to help "the least of these," the down trodden, helpless, hopeless, the sick, the lost, orphans, came bubbling to my surface the second I landed on that continent. There were so many who needed help that I knew instantly what I was designed to do. It is who I am, who God created me to be. As I worked with both short-term and career missionaries, I wondered if I, too, should be a career missionary. After all, I loved Africa, and wouldn't a devoted Christian be willing to spend her life— and not just a few months—helping those most in need?

After talking with many career missionaries, praying, and listening to my heart and soul and gut, I recognized that continuing short-term missions is what God was calling me to do. There clearly is a need for both. When I look back, I realize how distorted my view of Christ was—that I allowed myself to think that my worth was based on how much I did, not on who I was (and am).

I returned to work in urgent care and my comfortable life in the Twin Cities. Eventually, though, I became restless, especially when I considered how much I had taken for granted. The first time I walked into a grocery store after my inaugural trip to Africa was overwhelming; the lights, aisles, refrigeration, and overabundance of food. Oh, my goodness. My apartment was bigger than I needed, and the clothes in my closet could clothe many Kenyans. There was even a time when I felt like selling everything I had, until I realized that doing so meant that I would no longer be in a position to help in Africa.

I found it was harder to adjust to life in the U.S. after being in Kenya than first adjusting to Kenya. As time went on, I learned that if I wanted to live in both worlds, which was my calling, I had to separate my two lives. When I was in Africa, I learned to work within the resources available and not go ballistic with the lack of resources. On the other side of the coin, when I was in the U.S., I became less judgmental, recognizing that most people in America have no idea what it is like in underserved countries, so I can't expect them to have my same vision and passion. Okay, I admit, it took several years to learn this to the point of not going just a bit crazy.

I knew it was past time for me to return to Africa when I was no longer seeing our affluence, and was, once again, becoming comfortable in it. At that point, I needed Africa probably more than it needed me. So I called the mission I was working with to see if I could return to Tenwek Hospital. Hope said, "Yes, we can always use you at Tenwek, but where we really need you right now is in Somalia." Pause. Deep breath. I said, "Isn't there a war going on in Somalia right now?" She replied, "Yes, Susan. That's why we need you there." Hmmm. Another conundrum. I was ready to go back to Kenya where I knew I was relatively safe. But Somalia? During a war? "I'll get back to you, Hope. I need to do some more praying." That was a huge understatement. I knew God was calling me back to Africa; however, did that include a war zone? I had to make sure. So I prayed, read the Bible, did devotions, talked to people I trusted. I decided God was still calling me to Africa, and that meant Somalia. So I made a call, determined my departure time, and purchased tickets. I was set to go.

That was, until my dad had a heart attack, two weeks before my scheduled departure. *Now what is God trying to tell me?* Talk about trying to discover hope in the unexpected! Surely I couldn't go to the other side of the world where I would have no communication shortly after my dad's cardiac bypass surgery. Think of the continuing stress I would be putting on his triple bypassed heart! At least it happened before I left so I could cancel the trip rather than being out of touch in Mogadishu, Somalia. So I canceled. But something didn't feel right. It's my dad! Africa is calling. But my dad! The next week I went to a Lenten service and heard the verse Luke 9:59-60: "To another He said, 'Follow Me.' But he said, 'Lord, first let me go and bury my father.' But Jesus said to him, 'Let the dead bury their own dead; but as for you, go and proclaim the kingdom of God.'" Wow. Right between the eyes, there in black and white and red, not much interpretation needed. As I fought back tears, I left the church and went back to the hospital knowing what I had to do.

My parents were not surprised, but they also were not excited. They have always said I strengthen their prayer life. When I told my older sister, Kathy, a pastor and excellent preacher, she said, "Susan, you can't take Scripture so literally!" Two weeks later than initially planned, I was on a plane to Mogadishu, Somalia. Something I now recognize as the Holy Spirit tugged at me to go to church that random Wednesday night. I needed clarity on an answer that was evading me, and even though the text did not literally pertain to my situation, I had clarity.

Landing in Mogadishu, Somalia, was surreal. As we were taxiing down the runway after landing, the Indian Ocean was to our right, and to our left were gutted out buildings, army

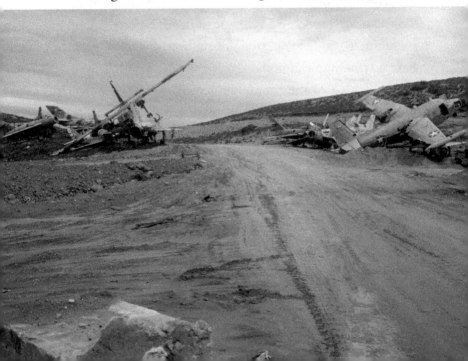

tents with various flags representing different countries, and men with guns. Many men with many guns. There wasn't really an airport, just an area with three walls and a roof that once was an airport. There were pieces of planes scattered everywhere—more signs of the war. What in the world was I doing here? Kenya was calling, I was sure of it. Again, I was proven wrong.

Somalia really *was* calling. When I arrived at our house, I learned that the team had been fervently praying for a physician to come at the time I arrived because they would have been down to one physician, an 80-year-old man. He held the wisdom I had not yet acquired as I provided the stamina, which in him was dwindling.

The moment I arrived back in the States, I started making arrangements to return in the fall to stay in Somalia for six months. These people were definitely people in need and there was no other doctor for them on the horizon. How could I not go back? How could I deny my passion and calling to help?

After three months back in Somalia, we were forced to leave. World Concern lived down the street from us and was bombed. Members of Save the Children UK were ambushed on the streets of Mogadishu and killed. We became targets and, after much prayer and discussion, decided that God was not calling us to be martyrs. We packed up and left for Nairobi, Kenya, on a gigantic Russian jet. Grace, Kia, and I were the only passengers with Russian pilots who did not speak English. Jim was staying a couple of extra days to wrap up loose ends. We sat on pull-down seats along the side of the plane. There was no cargo except our luggage, which looked tiny and lonesome at the tail end of the plane.

I still had three months before I was to return home and was asked if I would be willing to help in Southern Sudan. (At the time, Southern Sudan had not yet become an independent country.) My answer, of course, was *yes*. I remember in seventh grade geography we were to pick a country in Africa and write a report. Immediately, Sudan stood out to me and was, in my mind, the only option. "Sudan, Susan, how could I go wrong?!" After my first time in Kenya, Sudan frequently entered my mind. Eventually I said, "Okay God, if I ever am asked to go to Sudan I know it will be your call." So, I was off to Sudan from Somalia for three months! Or, so I thought.

One day, after being in Southern Sudan for two and a half months (two weeks before my scheduled departure to start my trek home to the States), I truly thought I was going to die. Men from a rival tribe came through our village on a cattle raid, randomly shooting anyone who got in their way. Since we had a UN flag flying over our compound, we were sure they would come for us, knowing they would find food and medicine. We waited three hours for a plane to evacuate us to Lokichokio, Kenya, the UN base for all work being done in Southern Sudan (Operation Lifeline Sudan). Miraculously, we survived. We later learned that 24 people from our village were killed that day.

A year after returning home from Southern Sudan, I knew I was being called again. My whole family knew. I remember a call from my sister, Beth, asking me when I would be leaving. After all, Rwanda was at war. As you may remember, my arrival in Rwanda was suffocating and anxiety producing, which led me to Nairobi, Kenya, for about a week. When I returned to Rwanda, the pit in my stomach was gone and anxiety much reduced, but I was always on high alert. And I mean always. I don't think I slept the entire time there. You're right, that's impossible. However, I didn't sleep well. Sleeping in a tent with machetes being the weapon of choice did not bring me comfort. We heard women wailing all night and didn't know why. Were they hurt, grieving, frightened, or experiencing the presence of Satan? This sounds harsh, but is honest—at the time, I did not want to know. People would say, "Don't look for Satan in hell, he's in Rwanda." They were absolutely right.

My friend Karen and I did whatever we could to help. We worked in the emergency room. We swept and cleaned dirty

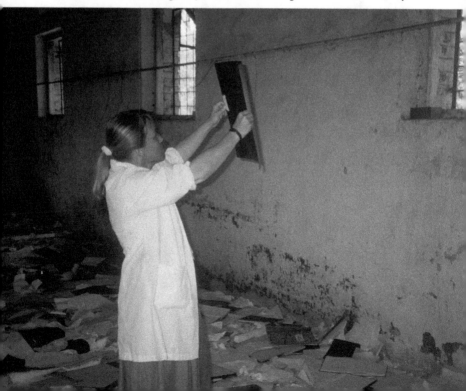

hospital rooms filled with discarded x-rays, papers, needles, broken vials. You name it, we swept it. Science fiction became real when we discovered there was a time warp at the hospital. Seriously. My watch would say 10:00. At least an hour later, I looked again, and it was 10:05. The days would never end! In Rwanda anything was possible, and the time warp felt as real as breathing.

But I couldn't leave. God was calling me to be a light in the darkness. This became evident the day I met Benwah. It was just him and me in the semi-secluded hospital grounds where I had taken a walk to pass the time. He looked to be about three or four years old, one of his legs was missing, and in its place was a sawed-off table leg. When he looked up at me, I was momentarily struck motionless. His smile was the most gorgeous thing I had seen in a very long time and lit up his whole body! I sat down on a cement step so I could look him in the eyes at his level while I smiled back. Immediately, he crawled into my lap and snuggled right in as I put my arms around him.

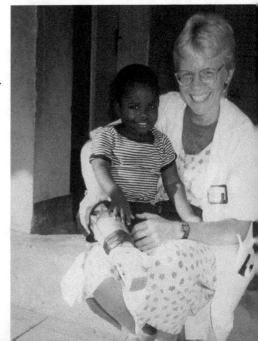

He had no intention of leaving and I had nowhere to be except right there. This was one time I didn't mind the time warp. I don't know how long we sat there (I had given up on the whole time thing), motionless, with his entire body curled into my lap except his wooden leg that didn't bend.

Eventually, a UN soldier walked by, looked at the scene and gave us his own big smile and said to me, "Benwah was found in an outlying village amongst his dead family members by a UN soldier who couldn't believe Benwah was alive; he had lost so much blood from his leg being cut off with a machete. The soldier brought him here to the hospital and then returned to his post. The soldier had blonde hair just like you. This is the first time I've seen Benwah let someone hold him." A light in the darkness. God was able to use me to provide a young boy a safe place, engulfed in love because I have blonde hair . . . and a vocation.

Several months after returning from Rwanda, the mission called and said they needed me to leave for Bosnia in a week. I said I needed two weeks. Bosnia-Herzegovina was at war with Serbia. Now I was forced into accelerated prayer, Bible reading, and discussion mode. I had been living my life devoted to daily quiet time with the Lord between mission adventures, so discernment didn't take as long. I was living my passion. I was ready for Bosnia!

In my mind, God and I had a great thing going! I worked urgent care nine months a year, which allowed me to go wherever He called me for three months a year. What an arrangement! I mean, not every doctor was willing to go to war zones, so it wasn't like someone else would fill in my overseas spot if I wasn't available. Not only was I fulfilling my calling and passion by working on both sides of the ocean, I enjoyed and embraced it! Surely God would not do anything to change this master plan of ours. Well, He only sees the master plan, His plan. The one in my head was just that, "mine" and not "ours."

While in Bosnia, doing the Lord's work I might add, my world was turned upside down. I was working in Hadzici, just outside of Sarajevo, during the transition between the signing of the Dayton Peace Accord and the time when the Serbs needed to vacate the communities they had taken over during the war. When we (a team of six) arrived, Sarajevo was like a ghost town with barricades everywhere and signs on street corners that read, "pazi snajper" (beware sniper).

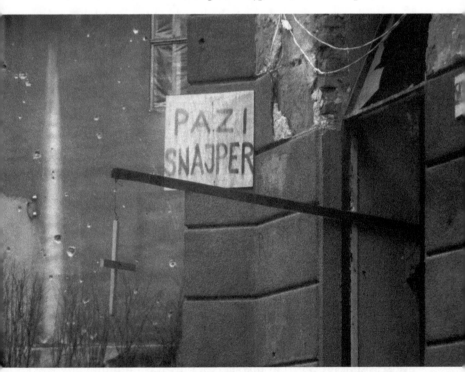

While disputing the outcome between two rival groups in Tarcin, a village in Hadzici, during the war with a lot of shooting all around, I injured my knee. That may be a little melodramatic for describing a basketball game, but it is all true. I injured my right knee while playing basketball. So I flew home alone with my luggage, a long leg cast, and the only pair of crutches in Sarajevo.

The following two years, in a nutshell (albeit a large nutshell), consisted of three knee surgeries, physical therapy, occasional work in urgent care, diagnosis of Complex Regional Pain Syndrome, multiple sympathetic nerve blocks to help the constant pain, a grand mal seizure when my aorta was inadvertently nicked during a nerve block, medicine with a side effect of gaining weight just by looking at food, and placement of a dorsal column stimulator (DCS) three times, which ultimately made my pain manageable and I no longer wanted my leg amputated. I was ready to move forward with life.

A week later, I received a letter from my employer stating my job was terminated and I was put on disability. Due to my limited mobility, I was also unable to do disaster relief overseas. What? Are you kidding me? God, what are You thinking!? We had such a good thing going and You are messing it all up! What am I supposed to do now?

Silence. Into the desert I went, feeling I had no purpose in life, alone, lost. I had been through a lot in my life; however, this was the most challenging yet. For the first time, I felt abandoned by God. The only way I remained spiritually intact was by listening to Christian music, a lifeline offered by God when I had nothing else to hold onto.

Finally, after two long years, I saw some light! My phone was ringing! (I understand that you can't really see a phone ring, but you also can't hear a light so just go with the imagery.) A Christian organization called to ask if I would be willing to help develop a children's heart program for children from countries that did not provide heart surgery. Children would be brought to the U.S. for surgery and then sent home after recovery. Hallelujah! My spark, which had basically become a pilot light burning only enough to not be snuffed out, was reignited. They could only pay me a small stipend and I would have to move across the country but, hey, at least I was on a path out of the wilderness.

Three years into the job, I knew I had to resign. I was physically, emotionally, and spiritually drained. Helping the children was fantastic and is what kept me going as long as I did. One weekend while visiting my sister, Kathy, she took one look at me and said, "Susan, you need to resign. If not, this job will kill you." She was right. It had become a job, and I was fighting for it to return to the passion and calling I felt the first couple of years. Physically, traveling became more difficult due to my knee pain, and sleep deprivation affected every aspect of my life. Emotionally, I was beat down by an organization that does wonderful things around the world but at the administrative level, it was an extremely difficult place for a professional woman to work. My role as a woman who is to be submissive to men came before my role as an administrator to the children's heart program. Eventually, all of this ate away at my spiritual life as I was living in a state of confusion. I was surrounded by Christian people working to help those most in need, so I wondered why I was so miserable. My sister saw what I could not see and pulled me out before I was snuffed out.

CONCEPT 2

God, what are You doing? You can't be thinking clearly! Why give me hope and then beat me down again? Silence. Back to the wilderness. Back to hanging onto the thread of Christian music that kept me breathing. After wandering a few months, I was talking with my psychologist and we focused on what I *had* rather than what I had *lost*. My intellect was still intact, so I needed to find a way to use that within my physical limitations.

Three weeks later, I sustained a traumatic brain injury (TBI). I couldn't believe it. Once I regained enough mental capability to realize my situation, I became livid. God, are You kidding me? Is this a joke to You? I'm not laughing. If You're trying to teach me something, please at least give me a hint. This is ridiculous! Why are You taking away my vocation, calling, mission, passion, and allowing my fire to slowly turn to ashes?

Silence. Back to the wilderness I went, struggling to keep my sanity, hanging onto my thread of music. After the TBI, I had difficulty putting words together to make a sentence. This added to my aloneness. I couldn't pray. Why bother? A friend told me to try to find a place where I could sit and imagine God's arms wrapped around me. What saved me was my Christian music and my hammock chair, the one place I felt God's presence—His arms firmly, yet softly, wrapped around me. I went to that place continually, music playing all the time. Sometimes the music was so quiet, I could barely hear it. It didn't matter. I was again infusing goodness into my brain, consciously and subconsciously.

REDIRECTING

I would like to make it clear that I don't believe God actively causes us pain and suffering. Rather, He allows the path that is set out before us in our sinful world. He grieves with us when we are in pain and promises to be with us through it all. My reaction was visceral, during my times of questioning God's presence when I felt my life was falling apart. Even though I knew He didn't cause it, why did He even allow all this to happen? When I am not wandering in the desert, I realize how truly blessed I am.

Shane and Shane are brilliant Christian musicians who I have enjoyed since their CD "Carry Away" came out in 2003. Shane Barnard is a master of lyrics and Shane Everett brings humor, an amazing tenor voice, and keeps Shane B on his toes. One of their songs, *Vision of You*, is the ringtone on my phone that I use for my alarm. I've heard these same words a million times, but it was just recently that one line hit me with its intended meaning. In fact, prior to my revelation, I thought it was a touch redundant.

Awaken what's inside of me
Tune my heart to all You are in me
Even though You're here, God, come
And may the vision of You be the death of me
And even though
You've given everything, Jesus, come

—Shane and Shane, *Vision of You*

This is just a portion of the song. The line, "Even though You're here, God come" initially sounded to me like it was repeating the same sentiment. However, during the writing of this book, as I'm more tuned in to everything around me, I finally understood the lyrics! God is always here. We can't go anywhere to escape Him since He is everywhere. Psalm 139: 7-10, "Where can I go from Your spirit? Or where can I flee from Your presence? If I ascend to heaven, You are there; if I make my bed in Sheol, You are there. If I take the wings of the morning and settle at the farthest limits of the sea, even there Your hand shall lead me, and Your right hand shall hold me fast."

So why do we have to invite Him in? Because He wants to be part of our inner circle when we're in community with each other, and He wants to be invited in to the core of our being when we are alone. During my days in the wilderness, God was with me, even though I did nothing to acknowledge His Presence. I thought He was being silent, not hearing my pleas of frustration and anger, and yet He was there all the time, feeling my pain, speaking through music. My heart's desire is to pray continually for Jesus to be the most integral part of my life, giving over all of my control to Him, recognizing His constant Presence in my life.

Today, my vocation is still medicine and helping those most in need. It looks a whole lot different than I ever imagined, but I still find ways to ignite my spark, even though my challenges continue. My vocation has been a moving target, and I don't see that changing any time soon. Thankfully, my medical knowledge was not affected by my TBI (I passed the Family Medicine Board recertification test the year after my injury);

however, I cannot keep up with the pace of U.S. medicine. I am still licensed and board certified, which means I can still make house calls and give advice and prescriptions. One huge blessing is being the road doctor for several Christian musicians. If they get sick while on tour, they contact me for advice and treatment. I see this as a way I can help the people who, through their gift of music, have given life to me for so many decades.

In addition, I am the Central African Republic (CAR) Partner Advocate for Global Health Ministries and have traveled to CAR several times to help expand public health education. I first traveled to Jamkhed, India, to learn about Community Based Primary Health Care (CBPHC). War has kept me out of CAR for the past several years, but I plan to return when some semblance of stability occurs.

When I fly to CAR, I go through Nairobi, Kenya, to help a dear friend, Robyn Moore, a nurse practitioner who has been living out her calling her entire life. We first met at Tenwek Hospital in 1990 when she was a pediatric nurse. She now has furthered her education and works in several orphanages with orphans and vulnerable children, a special needs center, and schools located in poor and high-risk areas. She is the definition of someone living out her passion, calling, and vocation by being exactly who God created her to be.

There are many ways we can live out our vocation in simple things we do, if we take the time to see past the routine and ordinary and grab opportunities that drop at our feet. Whatever our vocation is, showing love is a way to live it. Twenty years after my knee injury and 14 years after my TBI,

I still struggle. My abilities to process information and multitask are challenged, I fatigue easily, I move slowly. Love, I can do.

God is constantly molding us into being more like Him. Whatever is good in my life is God's doing; whatever is sinful is on me. My deepest desire is to get out of God's way so that when people see me, they see Jesus. Despite failing over and over, I want to live a life that reflects the life Jesus lived, helping the least of these wherever they cross my path, in my community or across the world. I want to live a life where I don't exist, just God in me. We are called to be open to what God is doing in our lives by living in close relationship to Him. Jesus will always have our back. Galatians 2:19-20: " . . . I have been crucified with Christ; and it is no longer I who live, but it is Christ who lives in me. And the life I now live in the flesh I live by faith in the Son of God, who loved me and gave Himself for me." I truly hope you are hearing that your life matters, right now and always.

Consider Moses. What a packed life of struggles, triumphs, challenges, hope, and defeat! First of all, he was to be killed at birth by the king of Egypt. Moses was an Israelite and the dictator king was in the process if thinning out the number of Israelites by killing all newborn boys in order to increase the Egyptian population. The mother of Moses, willing to give up her child to save his life, put him in a basket, and set him floating in the Nile River. Pharaoh's daughter found the baby and claimed him as her son.

Moses killed an Egyptian, fled to live with Israelites, married, and settled down in their land. The king of Egypt died, the

Israelites groaned under their slavery, and they called to God for help. God answered their pleas through Moses.

Moses was skeptical as can be at the start of his new vocation—but he freed the Israelites from bondage in Egypt and delivered them through the wilderness to the Promised Land.

First, Moses comes upon what appears to be a burning bush, but the bush is not burning, despite the flames. Through the burning bush, the Lord explains to Moses that he will deliver the Israelites from Egypt. Like many of us, Moses comes up with all sorts of reasons why this is a bad idea:

"Who am I that I should be the one?" said Moses.

"I will be with you and as a sign I will bring you back to this mountain when you escape," said the Lord.

"What if they ask me Your name?" said Moses.

"I Am who I Am," said the Lord.

"What if they don't believe me?" said Moses.

The Lord said, "Throw your staff on the ground." When Moses did, it turned into a snake. The Lord continued, "Pick it up by the tail."

When Moses did, it returned to a staff. God added one more miracle by having Moses put his hand in his pocket and when he brought it out, it was leprous. When he put it back in and out again, it was healed.

God said, "Do these miracles and if they still don't believe you, I'll give you a third. Pour water from the Nile on the ground and it will become blood."

Moses said, "But God, I can't speak well."

"I will be with your mouth and teach you what to say," said the Lord.

"Oh my Lord, please send someone else," said Moses.

The Lord intervened, giving grace to Moses, and told him his brother Aaron would help him and "even now he is coming to meet you . . . You shall speak to him and put the words in his mouth and I will be with your mouth and with his mouth, and will teach you what you shall do. He indeed shall speak for you to the people; he shall serve as a mouth for you, and you shall serve as God for him. Take in your hand this staff, with which you shall perform the signs," (Exodus 4:15-17).

Moses had no more to say—rather, obey.

> *You will be safe in His arms*
> *'Cause the hands that hold the world*
> *Are holding your heart*
>
> *This is the promise He made*
> *He will be with you always*
> *When everything is falling apart*
> *You will be safe in His arms*

—Phil Wickham, *Safe in His Arms*

CONCEPT 3

Search for an Unexpected Route

***

Be the wheels not the track
Be the wanderer that's coming back
Leave the past right where it's at
Be more heart and less attack

Ever growing, steadfast
And if need be, the one that's in the gap
Be the never turning back
Twice the heart any man could have

—NEEDTOBREATHE, *More Heart, Less Attack*

As my mathematician brother, Steve, would say, "Think outside the quadrilateral parallelogram." Steve is a brilliant mathematician and musician. He can calculate the square root of any number inside his head; he plays multiple instruments and has perfect pitch. When he was four years old, he asked my mom her age. He left the room briefly, returned, and announced her age in years, months, weeks, and days.

REDIRECTING

The next year, my sisters and I were in our basement watching the Olympics. We were more than surprised to hear the Olympic theme song being played on the piano upstairs. We looked at each other, knowing our parents were gone. Who could be playing the piano? "Where's Steve?" we all said at once. We raced upstairs, turned the corner into our living room, and saw our five-year-old brother sitting at the piano playing that theme song with both hands, sounding identical to what we had just heard on television. We were stunned! First of all, how did he get up on the piano bench? He was quite awkward with his legs and arms, but could do anything with his hands. He finished the song, looked at us with a smile, wiggled off the piano bench, and ran off.

Steve went on to finish college with honors in music and mathematics. Unfortunately, he can't maintain a job. My brother has autism. It took him six years and a lot of help to make it through college, but he did it! Now what? Good question. All of us are unique; however, in my opinion, the range of uniqueness of people on the Autistic Spectrum Disorder (ASD) is wider than any other subgroup of people I know. Hence the saying, "If you have met one person with autism, you have met one person with autism." In fact, that is why the new diagnostic term was needed for autism—ASD—which exemplifies the diversity. Thinking outside of the box is crucial to survival for people with autism and the community surrounding and supporting them. Thankfully, there are advancements being made that enable adults with autism to be part of the workforce by creating jobs that fit within their skills and accommodate their weaknesses. But doing so requires out-of-the-box thinking. For my brother and those in his situation, I hope and pray this work "accelerates exponentially," as Steve would say.

Unfortunately, we currently live in a society where many jobs are run by policies and procedures that can only be changed if a better way is scientifically or experientially (proven by experience) shown to be better. Some traditions are viewed as so absolute that change is not even an option. What would help is more creativity, flexibility, and people thinking outside the box.

Some great examples of thinking outside the box come from a very primitive area in Southern Sudan. Try to imagine Ulang, the village I called home for more than two months. Since my first view of Ulang was from the plane, I'll give you a bird's eye view. The village is spread out along the meandering Sobot River, providing the only water source for miles upon miles. Along the riverbank are canoes cut out of tree trunks, men fishing with nets, and women washing their children while others are swimming and laughing.

Sitting along the shore are a handful of men watching for crocodiles and snakes. Beside the river and running inland are tukels (mud huts) with grass roofs that are cut in unique

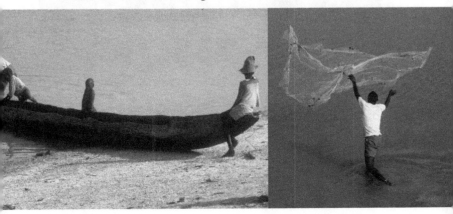

ways to make them look different from one another. Imagine someone with hair covering the full 360 degrees around his head, cut shoulder length. If you are old enough to remember the TV show "The Addam's Family," think of Cousin Itt. Now imagine that head to be in the shape of a cone. You are given a pair of scissors and told you can cut the hair any way you like with two exceptions. First, the innermost layer must remain shoulder length. Second, there must be no bald spots. In other words, you'll be making layers, which is what various grass roofs looked like.

Occasionally, you will notice that fences are used to divide the village into neighborhoods. Out of character are two sets of cement buildings, each unique, with openings for doors and windows. Meandering through the village are cattle, women and children carrying water in containers on their heads, men sitting making fishing nets or playing games in the dirt, and the elderly smoking long pipes.

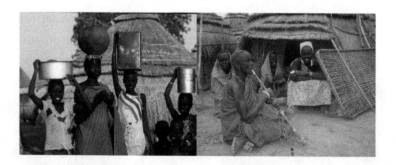

What stands out the most is a grass fence surrounding several green military tents, sand bags covering a bomb shelter, and a blue UN flag flying over the entrance. One of those tents was my home, shared with my friend, Kia Channer, who came with me to Sudan from Somalia.

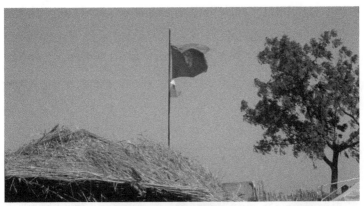

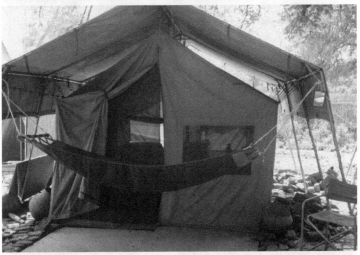

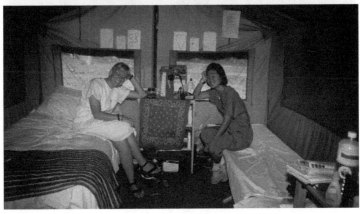

REDIRECTING

Now, imagine a quick walking tour of the Ulang Health Center. As we approach the health center, we see a rectangular grass fence with a "door" made from a plank of wood.

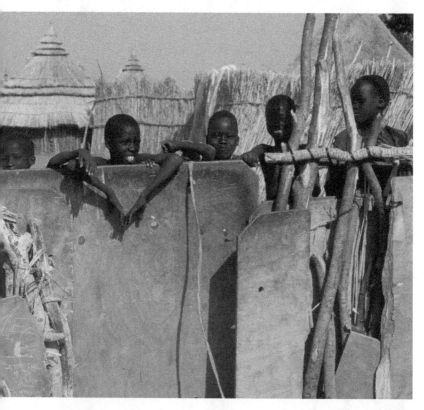

(If you remember the old westerns, think about half a saloon door.) As we enter the compound, in the center is one of the cement buildings we saw from the air, which is the clinic. The clinic has three rooms with doorways that open onto a cement slab. There are no doors. One room is the pharmacy, another the exam room, the last a procedure room. As we step back outside of the clinic, we see the hospital, which is the area inside the fence. Some patients came from great distances and were sick enough to need daily attention.

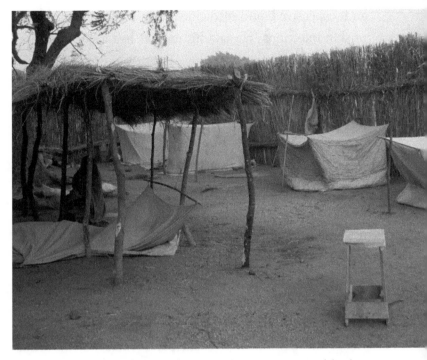

Any patient needing to stay overnight was given a blanket and mosquito net that they could set up within the fence. The Intensive Care Unit was a thing of beauty. In one corner within the Ulang Health Center fence was a grass roof. Yes, indeed. If someone needed IV fluids, they were put into the ICU where the IV bag could hang from the grass roof.

One would have to walk for days to find anything so advanced. The creation of the Ulang Health Center, better known as the clinic, was in itself thinking outside the box. The work done there and those touched by the center were absolutely a thing of beauty.

While at the clinic, I saw a young boy come into the procedure room every few days asking for Gentian Violet (GV), an inexpensive liquid medicine that is used for several types of skin infections. He said his mother had a skin infection, and he was treating it with GV. After a couple of weeks I said, through the translator, "I would love to visit your mother at your tukel to check her infection to see if there is something more we can do." He sheepishly looked down and his smile turned upside down as he said, through the translator, "My mother does not have a skin infection. I found a pen with no ink so I have been putting the purple stuff in my pen to write." Oh, my goodness. I put my arms around him and flashed him my biggest smile, which erased his frown. Pens were a hot commodity, which we passed out to the community health workers and traditional birth attendants to track patient visits. The only paper in the community was from the UN or us. Any other writing was done in the dirt. The village did have a single chalkboard. There was no formal education besides the little we provided. Not only had this young boy figured out a way to continue to write, but also found a source of paper. I didn't even ask where he obtained the paper. Rather, I kept filling his pen.

Initially, upon arrival in Ulang, I worked with the community health workers (CHWs) as a consultant. We would see patients together, and I would offer advice when asked and occasionally when I felt intervention was needed. Most CHWs have three months of training. We were blessed with one CHW who had 18 months of education. A couple of weeks after arriving in Ulang, I also was asked to work with traditional birth attendants (TBAs). Women's health was always handled by women, and since I was the first female physician to be in Ulang, it seemed a good time to help the

TBAs who had three months of training. Finding a translator was difficult because men wanted nothing to do with women's health, and it was the men who were educated and occasionally knew some English. On the many occasions when we did not have a translator, much of our communication was done through drawing pictures and hand gestures.

When I was informed the infant mortality rate the previous four months (when stats started to be recorded) was 90 percent, meaning nine out of 10 babies born died, the enormity of this responsibility weighed heavily on me. How could it not? Imagine living in a community where only one out of 10 babies born survived. It was difficult for me to wrap my head around.

When I first met with the two TBAs and their assistant, I learned how they delivered babies, what resources were available, and asked how I could best help them. In my experience, one mistake Americans tend to make is to go into other countries and tell them how they ought to change what they are doing and then proceed to tell them how to do it our way. There is much more success when the Nationals (local people) are involved from the beginning and are given the major role in decision making. I have always been of the mindset that when going into a different culture, it is best to ask a lot of questions and listen before giving my own opinions. Such was the case with the TBAs and their assistant. We were a comical looking bunch as we exchanged information in whatever manner we could, whether that meant using pictures, hand gestures, or demonstration. I often felt I was playing a game of Charades. Thankfully, the head TBA knew a few, and I mean *few*, English words. When they showed me the kit they used when delivering a baby, I was impressed. For those of you who help put together midwife kits that are distributed around the world, I say thank you. They are put to good use. I asked the TBAs to notify me when the next delivery happened so I could watch.

Late one evening, I was beckoned to a tukel and arrived just after a baby boy had been delivered. Everything appeared to have gone well. The child was lying in his mother's lap as the TBA was encouraging the mother to start breastfeeding. The only thing that seemed odd was the demeanor of the mother, who appeared a bit detached. Otherwise, mother and baby looked good, so I went back to bed. I knew this little boy would be one of the 10 percent who survive. On my way to the clinic the next morning, I stopped by the tukel where I had been just a few hours earlier. I was not prepared for what I saw and heard.

The TBA was there explaining to the mother that her son was dead. What? That made no sense! Despite appearing detached after her son was delivered, she was now in tears being consoled by the TBA who had no answers to give this mother. The TBA looked at me for help, holding eye contact for a long time, until finally I gestured, "I don't know" and broke eye contact by looking at the ground. *I had no answers.* I was here to help them. What was I missing? A healthy baby boy is delivered in the evening and dead the next morning, and I had nothing to say. I went over the entire scenario in my mind trying to see something that was eluding me. Nothing came. But then it dawned on me. I was thinking like an American when I needed to be thinking outside the box, taking into consideration the circumstances surrounding me.

I replayed the evening in my mind. I left the tukel as the infant was breastfeeding. I went back to my tent and slipped under my covers to go to sleep. Wait a minute! *I slipped under my covers!* Could that be it? The hot season had not yet started, so nights cooled down enough for me to need a sheet and wool blanket to stay warm. My mind went back to my departing scene at the tukel. Now I saw what I had missed. The baby was still wet from the delivery, and the mother was wearing only a thin skirt. There were no blankets in the tukel. The baby died from hypothermia! Could that be the answer for all of the deaths? They were dying because they were too cold from being wet and naked? August was the end of the hot season, so it started to cool down in September, which is when infant births and deaths started to be tracked. I talked with the TBAs to see if they had anything to dry the babies after they were born. "No," they answered. This situation changed immediately. Each TBA was given a towel to dry the babies after they were born, wash it, and have it ready for the next delivery.

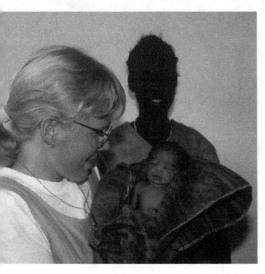

Next, I had to come up with a way to provide each baby with a blanket. Supplies were flown in every three to four weeks, which was too long to wait. There was no money system, much less a store. Hold on a second. We had blankets at the clinic to use for patients who stayed overnight. Where did those come from? The UN! I scrounged around for extra blankets and found 11.

We could cut one blanket into four pieces and give one to every newborn baby. In the month of January, there were 19 deliveries and only three deaths. All of the deaths occurred before we started using the towels and blankets. During the remainder of my time in Ulang, there was only one infant death who was very premature and needed oxygen, which we didn't have available. Even a set of twins were delivered and survived. Towels and blankets saving lives! I still get goosebumps.

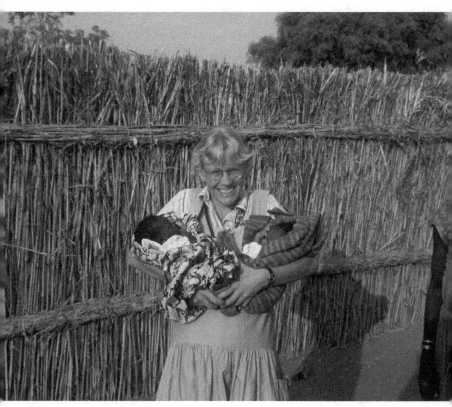

Thinking outside the box is a must no matter where we find ourselves. For instance, we used pill bottles to dispense liquid medicine to an individual patient. Cassava (manioc), a root made into a type of flour, was dried on the side of the road in Cameroon and CAR because the asphalt dried it quickly.

In Kenya, we found that an easy and inexpensive way to treat scabies, a skin infection caused by a mite that burrows under the skin, was to scrub the entire body with a corn husk and then wash with Omo bar soap, the only brand of soap available in the Tenwek Hospital area. At one point, when I was working at Tenwek, I had 58 patients in my 40 beds (the hospital averaged 110 percent occupancy), which occasionally required some creativity. For instance, one patient required her head to be elevated and another required her feet to be elevated. Hence, they shared a bed. Another time mandated an extravagant game of Operator: A patient from the Kisii tribe spoke only the Kisii language. The local language is Kipsigis, the national language is Swahili, and the international is English. My translator knew English and Kipsigis, but not Kisii. Thankfully, there was another patient from the Kisii tribe who spoke Kisii and Kipsigis but not English. Therefore, I spoke English to my translator who spoke Kipsigis to the one Kisii patient who then spoke Kisii to the first patient who only knew Kisii. Are you confused yet? Imagine my confusion when I would ask a question that went down the pipeline, the patient answered in great detail, the answer went back up the pipeline, and when it got to me the answer was one or two words. Talk about lost in translation! I'm confident that the message from God to Moses to Aaron to the people was not lost in translation!

REDIRECTING

The Sudanese can think outside the box like no other when it comes to fashion. They made good use of *everything*. My friends and family will attest to the fact that I have no fashion sense, so if I have to dress beyond jeans and a t-shirt, watch out. The people in Ulang taught me some tricks on how to do more with less. The vast majority of children had no clothes, but many were adorned with jewelry made from melted shell casings, beads, and string. The women typically wore a ragged thin skirt with no top. Most men had pants or shorts, usually with a shirt, or material they wrapped around their body. A few adults had no clothes. Since there was no money system, we bartered for what we wanted, which sometimes involved clothes, but usually pens. We tried to give clothes to those most in need. What impressed me about the people is that they preferred bartering over hand-outs, and if they had nothing to give in return, they immediately said a prayer of thanks for the generous gifts God provided. One such incident has been imprinted on my heart and mind forever.

One of the patients we were caring for was a young boy with kala azar (a parasitic infection spread by sand flies that slowly and painfully sucks the life out of the person).

His mother not only cared diligently for him, but also helped other patients who were too sick to care for themselves. All she had to wear was a ragged piece of cloth that she wrapped around her waist. One day, I gave her one of my dresses. As tears streamed down her face, she clasped my hands, looked to heaven, and offered a prayer of thanks. After her son died, she carried him for the three-day trek to her home village, buried him, and then made the three-day walk back to our clinic to continue helping the other patients.

CONCEPT 3

The Bible text for worship one Sunday in Ulang was from Luke 12:22-31. The first two verses: "He said to His disciples, 'Therefore I tell you, do not worry about your life, what you will eat, or about your body, what you will wear. For life is more than food, and the body more than clothing.'" I couldn't help but wonder what the Sudanese people were thinking about while hearing this passage. They *do not* have enough food and clothing, so it would appear that they *do* have to worry about what they will eat and what they will wear. Watching the faces of the people while they listened to this text made me realize how strong their faith is. They did not appear to be as bothered by these words as I was; rather, they were reassured and heard the promise that God will care for us. They were able to look beyond this present life toward the hope of an eternal life after death. I'm not saying they didn't care about the lack of food and clothing; instead, they seemed to accept it and did what they could to survive.

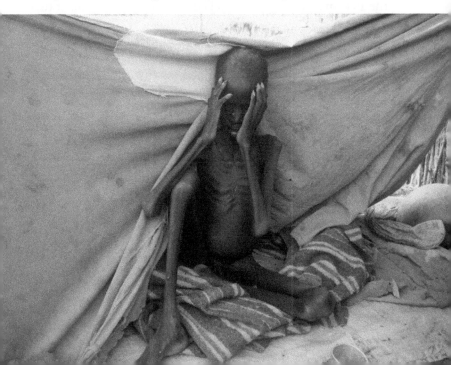

God has provided the world with enough food and clothing, and it is our responsibility to distribute them evenly. It was a humbling day.

One day, when a plane brought us supplies, included were several boxes of donated clothes, which were to be dispersed in Ulang. Most of the clothes were very old fashioned, but the people in Ulang were not aware of fashion trends. The clothes were distributed by the local officials, so these leaders came into our compound and split them up amongst themselves, then left with their bundles to start the general distribution. Watching them was like watching kids in a candy store. They were so excited!

The fun really started for us the following day. Like the first day of school, people were wearing their "new" clothes for all to see. Kia and I were entertained by the fashion show. The first man we saw was decked out in his new pink tutu, appearing ready to jump on stage for the ballet, clueless as to the garment's real purpose. Just beyond the man in the tutu, we saw a boy of about five years walking in our direction. The smile on his face was absolutely radiant. He was overjoyed because he had his first pair of socks!

And it was not only his first pair of socks; it was his first piece of clothing apparel, period. He was as proud as could be with his pair of green socks! The fact that they had no elastic left in them made no difference to him. He would take a couple of steps, stop to pull up his socks, take a couple more steps, stop to pull up his socks—always with a smile as stunning as can be.

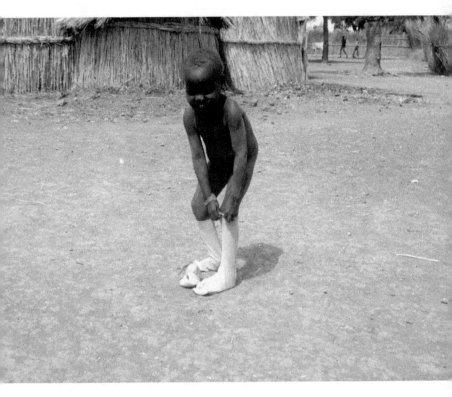

People were inventive—a quality reflected in many ways, including the fashioning of incredibly creative hats. One day, a woman came into the clinic wearing a pair of training pants on her head. Since the Sudanese do not have diapers or training pants of any sort, she thought they must be a hat. I discovered just about anything can be used as a hat. Some hats were made out of old boxes, burlap, or whatever else could be found. We found we had to be very careful about what we threw away. We burned all of our garbage, but there were times our scraps were rummaged through before we could burn them. In fact, it wasn't surprising to see some of our discarded items on someone's head. One day, I noticed a child wearing an empty blue and white Goody's box on his head.

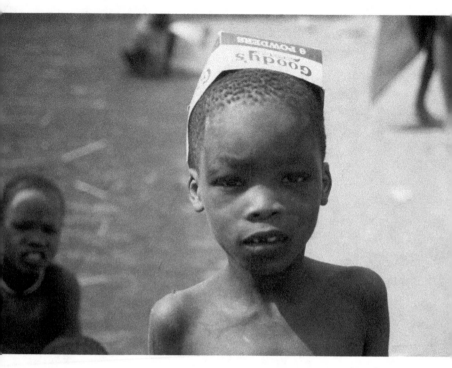

I had thought that the sole purpose of the box was to store Goody's headache powder. This child had resurrected the box for a whole new purpose. Surgical masks, it turns out, also make lovely hats.

Clothes were also very creative. Often, they were made of scraps of material sewn together in all sorts of ways, reminding me a bit of the Biblical story describing Joseph's coat of many colors. I must admit that the most intriguing fashion statement was worn by two girls the day after a food drop. They collected the plastic and rope that had been around boxes of food supplies dropped from an airplane and made dresses from the plastic and belts from the rope. Not only were these outfits completely see-through, but they were as hot as the dickens.

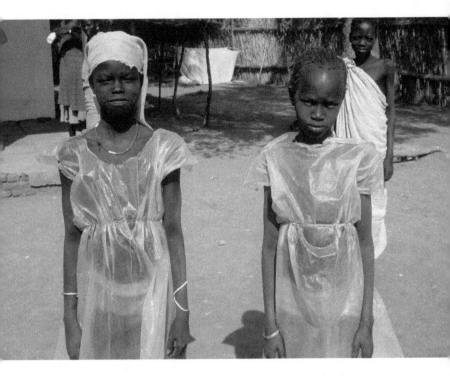

One Sunday morning as I was sitting in church, looking out into the sea of faces, I was struck motionless when I saw a small child wearing a full snowsuit!

The temperature was over 100 degrees F! Thankfully, the boy's mother did take the hood off about half way through the service. I was sweating just looking at him. For those of you who donate clothes to missions, keep sending snowsuits. Having been on the receiving end of a container sent to CAR by Global Health Ministries (GHM), I understand how difficult it is to organize what is put in a container for a specific location. Overall, everything sent was appropriate for our situation; however, sometimes an oddity is bound to appear. By thinking outside the box, everything is used.

REDIRECTING

In contrast to the heat, one of the quietest days in the clinic was the day a cold front moved through the village, keeping people inside their tukels and venturing out only in an emergency. These tukels were actually quite ingenious. In my ignorance, I had initially thought that the tukel was only a simple mud hut with the sole purpose of providing shelter. I soon learned differently. For instance, in the intense midday heat, I could step into a tukel where the air felt cool, but on a cool day, it was warmer inside than out. My tent had it backwards; on hot days it became even hotter inside the tent and vice versa.

As Kia and I were walking to the clinic on the day of the arctic air, we immediately noticed that the village appeared to be deserted. And then I saw, for the first time, an African dressed as an Eskimo. He was wearing a woman's coat with fur lined sleeves that barely reached his elbows, and a fur lined hood that was pulled down over his face and tied tightly, exposing only his eyes. But this was just the beginning. Upon arrival at the clinic, we saw a whole new fashion statement. Not only were men decked out in women's coats, but we saw a new line of winter hats—most notably wigs, mostly worn by men. One man in his 30s, around six-and-a-half feet tall, wore a red and black plaid women's wool coat that barely reached his thighs and elbows, and a wig with long brunette hair.

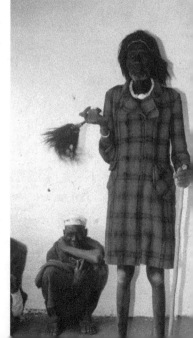

In retrospect, I realize that it was the men who had the warm clothes, and therefore were out and about in the village while the women and children tried to stay warm in their tukels. I guess the snowsuit wasn't such a bad idea. Interestingly, the temperature on that "wintry" day was around 82 degrees F, which came unexpectedly during the hot season. I know that doesn't sound much like an arctic front, but it makes sense when put into perspective. Usually the temperature was well into the 100s during the day, so 82 degrees was at least 20 to 30 degrees colder than usual. Picture yourself in the summer when the temperature has been 80 for a month. If you wake up one day and the temperature is below 60 degrees, it feels cold. On the other hand, if you have had a winter stretch with temperatures of 0 degrees, you feel warm if the temperature suddenly hits the 20s or 30s. Our bodies are amazing in infinite ways, one being the way we can adjust our comfort level to fit the climate.

One phenomenon that never ceased to amaze me was the fact that most people, especially children, shared the clothes they had. It was as though clothes were community property that could be used for a while and then turned over to someone else, much like a library book. Due to the limited supply, we knew the entire repertoire of clothes in the village and became accustomed to seeing a piece of clothing worn by someone different from the person we had seen wear it the day before. In fact, even though my wardrobe was predictable, it was luxurious in their eyes. After all, I had an unheard of three changes of clothes. Most people had so much less.

It reminds me of a woman who crawled into our compound one day while in Southern Sudan. She was struggling because she was crawling while trying to hold on to a table leg. Where she found that, we'll never know. The reason she was not walking was because her right leg below her knee was gone and had been for some time. Both of her knees were calloused and white from her years of crawling. She came to us asking if we could attach the table leg to her leg so she could walk again. Using ingenuity and whatever supplies he could find, Henry, a handyman, figured out a way to tie the table leg onto her leg, which also gave her the ability to remove it when needed. For the first time in many years, she stood up. She was even able to walk home!

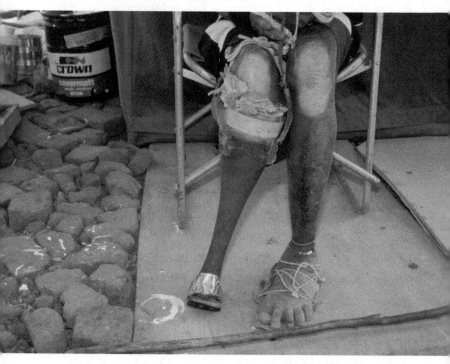

Survival and personal success come when we think outside the box. Like my Sudanese friends, I, too, have had to think outside the box so that I am able to follow my passion and live out my vocation. Has my path diverted? Of course. So now I keep my hands in medicine and help those in need in whatever way possible, taking advantage of the ordinary moments in life and grabbing opportunities in whatever way God leads. Much of this is done by paying attention to things around me that I have taken for granted or been too distracted to notice.

The power of being in the present as God is working through me is my vocation. I am living a life of meaning and purpose, and my new levels of availability have proven to be a blessing to many. Judy Siegle, a friend since college, is a quadriplegic motivational speaker and author. She cannot travel alone so I have the pleasure of being her travel companion, which benefits both of us.

These past two weeks alone, I was called upon by a neighbor who needed help replacing his antibiotic prescription while another neighbor needed her blood pressure checked. A friend called from work after suffering shortness of breath, a racing pulse, and chest discomfort. Even though he felt fine at the moment of the call, he was sure he was going to die. "Doc, what do I do? I feel fine now." I said, "Have someone drive you directly to the Emergency Room." Another friend, visiting relatives in another state, texted me a picture of her infected eye, which needed antibiotics, hence a phone call to a pharmacy. The next texts were regarding a bladder infection, an ear infection, and the need for a prescription for an anti-malaria medicine for someone heading off to Africa.

Then, another. This time closer to home. My 87-year-old dad, the very same man to endure the triple bypass prior to my trip to Rwanda, fell flat on his face, hitting his chest. These are situations where I go into medical mode, become focused, and push everything else out of my mind. His glasses left a gash under his right eye in the shape of a smile, classic for my dad, the eternal optimist, and a hematoma (mass of blood) was starting above his eye. The area surrounding his entire eye was already black and blue. My sister, Pastor Kathy, went into care-giving mode, which started with a quick prayer, while my mom turned on her inner caretaker. I got busy pulling the skin edges together with surgical tweezers, then after I put a sticky solution on his skin to keep them in place, Kathy applied the steri-strips. I asked my dad, "Do you hurt anywhere?" He said, "Around my eye. And my chest." Please, no. Not the answer I wanted. After more questions and an exam, I concluded it was costochondritis (inflammation along the sides of the sternum), not heart related. I love medicine! Not that I'm glad my dad was hurt, but that I was able to take care of him, that my vocation is tied to medicine, caregiving, and now, writing.

Sometimes living out our calling can have consequences beyond our control—both good and bad. Two years ago, I was asked if I would stay with Manny, the 14-year-old son of friends, Myrtle and Dave, who needed to be out of the country for two weeks. I agreed because I was available. Manny has signs of high-functioning autism, and because autism is close to my heart, we responded well to each other. I was happy I was available to help my friends. Some of my other friends thought I was being taken advantage of and should say no or require some kind of payment for my help. But that's not who I am. I was being given an opportunity to live out my calling, so why not?

Manny and I had a great time when he wasn't at school. He's a computer whiz and taught me so much; I felt I was in the 22nd century! He was calm and smiled more than I had ever seen. Unbeknownst to me, his step-brother, Clint, from Myrtle's first marriage, was also staying in the house, which became apparent to me only when I smelled marijuana smoke billowing from the family room. I told Clint, a 25-year-old man, that he could not use any drugs in the house. Thankfully, he found a friend who agreed to house him while his parents were away. Manny and I had a wonderful time together—that is until Myrtle and Dave returned home. Shortly after they arrived, Manny's older sister, Milly, and Clint returned to the house and a loud fight broke out in the attached garage. I instantly saw a change in Manny's demeanor. He closed in on himself, sat on a chair in the living room, trying to appear to do homework, his eyes giving away his fear as they kept shifting back and forth to the garage. Immediately, I went to him, knelt in front of him, and asked if he was afraid of the fighting. He nodded. I assured him that I would not leave until the fighting had stopped and his sister and step-brother were gone. He nodded, looked at me, and gave me a half grin. I knew his sister had threatened him multiple times in the past, so it did not take a genius to figure out he did not want to be left alone in this mess.

Eventually, Milly left and Dave, Myrtle, and Clint came in the house and sat at the dining room table. I joined them. Myrtle and Clint continued to have occasional outbursts, and because it felt like a potentially volatile environment, I stayed. Shortly after mid-night, Myrtle went to her bedroom and immediately fell into a deep sleep. Clint left through the front door. Since it was so late, I decided to sleep on the couch one more night. Before lying down, I took the dogs out, and went to the kitchen to fill their water bowls. Dave was coming into the kitchen as I was leaving, and we talked briefly. Within minutes, I saw Clint come out of nowhere behind Dave and hit him hard on the back of his head.

The next thing I knew, I was on my back trying to get up off the floor, but was struggling because a body was on top of me. As soon as I was halfway standing, something hit me and I was face down on the floor. Again, I was pushing against bodies, this time it felt like two bodies on top of me. I finally stood up, trying to shake some sense into my brain, when Clint looked me in the eyes like a deer caught in headlights. In his drug and drunken state, he did not realize I was even there. He said, "You saw him throw the first punch, right?" I shook my head and said, "No." He bolted from the kitchen and out of the house. I found my broken glasses, looked at Dave, and thought, "He's dead." He was unconscious, face down in a pool of blood spreading around his head. I found my phone, called 911, turned Dave over so he could start breathing. Thankfully, he did, as I was shouting for Myrtle to wake up. The paramedics arrived quickly and were able to get Dave talking. He had been unconscious for about 15 minutes. Dave was a volunteer firefighter and well known by the first responders. But he was nearly unrecognizable to them. His face was swollen and discolored.

Had I chosen not to follow my calling to care for Manny those two weeks, Dave would have been killed. Clint is now in prison for two felonies related to the assault. Both Dave and I had multiple broken bones among other injuries. Did the outcome affect how I would have made my original decision? No. I was being who God created me to be. That's vocation. That's a calling. That's our passion. It's not always easy.

Globally, mission work continues to evolve as we all think outside the box. Fifty years ago, we were more focused on building hospitals and clinics in underdeveloped areas and staffing them with missionaries from developed countries. This worked well for a while; however, it became harder to find people willing to spend their entire life in an underdeveloped country. Add to that the importance of Nationals feeling ownership and empowerment in their own lives. Slowly, mission has evolved to become more education-oriented with a focus on empowering people in underdeveloped areas to care for themselves. My most recent international mission work has me thinking outside the box since it is different than what I had ever done before.

I am learning about community-based primary health care, which is a template that I learned in Jamkhed, India, that focuses on four main points. First, equity, with a particular focus on serving the poorest of the poor. Second, integration, including food and animal production, water, sanitation, education, health care, and economic development. Third, empowerment of individuals and communities that places a high priority on empowerment of women as the main protectors of health for children and families. Fourth, appropriate technology (technology that is locally available, repairable, can be operated with irregular power supplies in humid or dry conditions, and can be used with minimal training). As

REDIRECTING

I said earlier, I am currently the Central African Republic Partner Advocate for Global Health Ministries. It is all about empowerment and the immeasurable benefits of thinking outside the box.

Tenwek Hospital in Kenya is one more example of out-of-the-box thinking. It started in the 1930s basically as a dispensary and grew into a clinic and hospital run by nurses. The first doctor, Ernie Steury, arrived in 1959. Over the decades, Tenwek Hospital has gradually evolved from an American-run clinic and hospital to a Kenyan-run clinic and hospital with Americans helping more in consulting and teaching roles. They started a nursing school that feeds well-trained Kenyan nurses into the hospital. Later, medical students and medical Residents from Nairobi rotated through Tenwek. Outreach includes outpost clinics, agriculture education, public health education, and more. Now many of the workers are Kenyan, from the top down, including the CEO. To make a lasting change such as this takes time. We don't always live to see the results of our toils.

Dr. Ernie Steury and Dr. Dave Stevens in 1984 had a conversation that redirected Tenwek's history. The hospital was dependent on a generator for electricity and was only able to run for 7-8 hours per day. As fuel prices rose, it became harder and harder to use it as often as they needed electricity. Next to the hospital is a river with a waterfall. Dr. Stevens was getting ready to go on furlough so Dr. Steury, half-jokingly, asked Dr. Stevens if, in addition to raising money to support his ministry, he would also raise money for a hydroelectric plant to generate energy from the waterfall. Three years later, the hydroelectric plant was up and running, revolutionizing the hospital and mission living quarters.

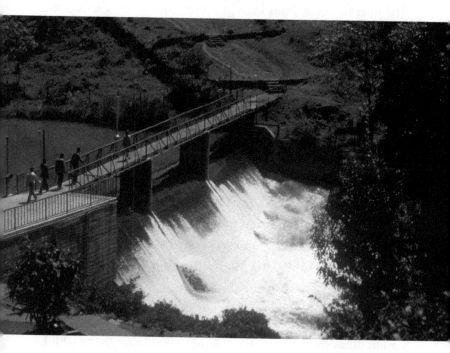

It can be frightening to think outside the box. Remember in the Old Testament when Joshua crossed the Jordan River with the Israelites? They had been wandering through the wilderness for 40 years and were finally going to Jericho and the Promised Land. The waters of the Jordan River didn't part like the Red Sea when Moses raised his staff. This time, God told Joshua he had to first step into the river followed by 12 priests carrying the Ark of the Covenant before He would part the river. What faith they must have had to step into the raging river, holding the Ark of the Lord, and get their feet wet before the river parted. Sometimes *we also* have to get our feet wet before the waters part.

REDIRECTING

If we really want to get down to out-of-the-box thinking, consider Jesus himself. The Pharisees wanted to keep Him in the box; however, Jesus kept jumping from inside the box to outside, on the edges, in the margins, on the fringe, outside of the fringe, everywhere inside and outside the box—but mostly outside the box. He healed on the Sabbath, which was unlawful, saying that the Sabbath was made for humans, not humans for the Sabbath. He said that those who want to save their life will lose it, and those who lose their life for Him would find it. Huh? Something to ponder. Also, a woman with an unclean reputation named Mary Magdalene and a scorned tax collector named Zacchaeus would become followers of Jesus, who accepted them with open arms. And how is it that this man who was crucified on a cross became Savior of the world? After His resurrection, He appeared first to women rather than the disciples or church leaders. That was totally outside the box!

Sometimes our calling takes us down paths we never could have imagined.

Oh, can anybody show me the real Jesus?
Oh, let Your love unveil the mystery of the real Jesus
Jesus started something new
Jesus coined a phrase or two
Jesus split the line at the turning point in time
Jesus sparked a controversy
Jesus, known for His mercy, gave a man his sight
Jesus isn't white

—Downhere, *Real Jesus*

CONCEPT 4

Relish the Journey as Much as the Destination

All that you're working for
Could blind you to
The treasures all around you
So don't miss these
Moments, please
The joy before
The crown you seek

Open your eyes
Your prize is right
Before you somehow
Whatever you do,
Just don't miss now

—Downhere, *Don't Miss Now*

There is something that happens to people who face death: It helps them to appreciate each day they're alive. And, while sometimes I can't even remember a single thing of significance that I accomplished the previous week, I do recognize that all of life is a journey, one step at a time. If any of you are like me, there has been a time in your past when you have said something like, "Coach, I know I didn't have a good practice, but I'll give 110 percent tomorrow." "Mom, I haven't practiced the piano all week, but next week I'll give 101 percent." This is mathematically impossible to do—giving more than 100 percent. If 100 percent means we're giving our all, then if we give more than 100 percent, we weren't giving our all when we thought we were at 100 percent. In other words, we can't give more than our all, which is 100 percent. My niece, Sarah, was four years old when the movie *Toy Story* was released. One night, I was putting her to bed and we were talking about how much we loved each other. It would end with, "I love you to infinity!" Since we had both seen the movie, I added, "I love you to infinity and beyond!" She pondered for a moment and then said, "If infinity means what I think it means, how can you go beyond infinity?" Good question. You cannot. Just as you cannot give more than 100 percent.

My point is that each moment is 100 percent important and cannot be taken back. In other words, life is a journey, not a destination. If we have our eyes too focused on the destination, we lose sight of being present in the moment.

I can't help but think about Monyon. As I was leaving our compound in Southern Sudan one morning, a small child quietly came to my side and walked next to me. He was about three or four years old, naked, with jet black skin made a lighter shade of gray with the dusting of dirt. His arms and legs were as thin as toothpicks, and his protruding stomach looked out of place with the rest of his skinny body. He would intermittently steal a glance up at me, and then look away when I looked down at him.

Despite being in a hurry to get to the clinic, I decided it was time to make an introduction. I got down on one knee, pointed to myself and said, "Susan." I then pointed to him and gave him an inquisitive look in an attempt to tell him that I wanted to know his name. It was then that I got my first glimpse of a smile that is forever imprinted on my mind. His smile showed missing front teeth—but lit up his entire face. He pointed to himself and said, "Monyon." I offered my hand to him and said, "Nice to meet you, Monyon." Of course, he had no clue what I said, but at the sound of his name he grabbed my hand and didn't let go until we reached the clinic.

As always, the clinic was very busy and both physically and emotionally draining. Each day, I left with a heavy heart. However, on this day, as I was leaving to head home, I found Monyon waiting for me. He flashed me a smile, took my hand, and walked me home. That was the first of my daily walks with Monyon, my own personal escort. No matter how weary I was at the end of a day, I could always look forward to my walk home with Monyon, who would light up the village with his smile.

One day, I went for a walk with Kia, the nurse who came with me

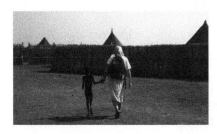

from Somalia to Sudan. We were quickly joined by Monyon and another three-year-old boy; they both clasped my hands and wouldn't let go.

REDIRECTING

Kia had one free hand, which was held by multiple children at various points of our walk. Monyon and his friend were the only two to stay with us for the entire walk. Children frequently rubbed the skin on my arms to see if it felt as strange as it looked—they had never seen skin so white. The adults were probably too reserved or polite to rub my arm, so they settled for shaking my hand when it was available.

We walked along the river, and when we got to the outskirts of town, we headed across a field toward the military compound—basically a building that housed a few weapons. It appeared abandoned, so I took my camera out to take pictures. We quickly learned that it was not abandoned when two men with guns ran out of the building. We did not need to know their language to understand that they were telling me to put my camera away and start walking in the other direction. We obviously did what we were told. Both boys were so quiet during the whole trek, and as we were heading back toward the village, I noticed that they were walking a little funny, as though they were tiptoeing on hot coals. I looked down, and both of them had feet full of little thorns. They hadn't complained at all, partly because they didn't want to risk stopping and giving up our hands. I felt so bad. Of course, I hadn't noticed the thorns, because I was wearing shoes. We stopped, pulled out the thorns, and continued our journey. I was humbled by their devotion to us.

One day, as I was leaving the clinic, Monyon was particularly animated and excited as he tried to take my backpack. I soon realized that he wanted to carry it home for me. I chuckled, shook my head, and said, "It is way too heavy for you, Monyon." Again, he had no idea what I was saying, but he loved hearing me speak his name. What he did not realize was that my backpack contained my medical bag, 35mm camera with attachments, books, and other things that made it weigh probably four times what he weighed.

I started walking as I had every other day, expecting him to take my hand. When he didn't, I looked down at him and could see pure determination on his face. I quickly realized that he was serious about this! I figured I could give him the backpack to carry for a few steps until it became too heavy. I took the backpack off of my back and slowly put his arms through the straps. I didn't want to let go completely because I was afraid he would topple over . . . and worse, bruise his pride. I kept holding the top of the pack to relieve some of the weight. However, Monyon would have none of that! He wanted to carry it by himself, and I was hurting his feelings by not showing him that I believed he could do it. I slowly let go of my grip. I still figured he would take it a few

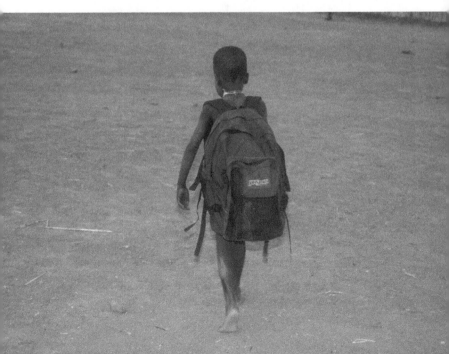

steps to show his act of kindness and then give it back to me. We walked a short distance, and I looked down at him and gave him my inquisitive look again to see if he was ready to give the pack back. He just smiled up at me and kept walking—and walking and walking. At one point he let go of my hand in order to use both his hands to help hold the pack. He started hunching over from the weight and was sweating profusely from the strenuous exercise. But he was determined to continue.

By the time we reached my tent, he was practically crawling, but he proudly attempted to stand up straight as he wiggled out from under the pack. I didn't think his smile could get any bigger, but I'm quite sure that it now literally went from one ear to the next. Although Monyon never again offered to carry my backpack, he continued to walk me home every day. It all started with being present in the moment the first day we met.

One difference I have seen between the United States and underdeveloped countries such as Southern Sudan and Central African Republic is that Americans oftentimes look to the future, whereas my African friends live for the present, one day at a time. We have the luxury of scheduling events for the next week, month, or year. They do not. In both Southern Sudan and CAR, their main goal when they wake each morning is to live through the day. Think about that for a moment. I understand there are people in the U.S. who, due to age or disease, also wake up with the hope of making it until tomorrow, and I don't want to diminish what they are experiencing. In fact, they are really the only ones who can relate to these Africans. Every day, people in Africa may ask the same questions over and over again. Will the water supply still have water? Will the fields be producing grain? Will war return destroying everything we have started to grow? Who will die from malaria today? I bring this up for a few reasons. First, to acknowledge how blessed we are. Second, to realize how much of a blessing we can be. And, third, so we never forget that the journey is as important as the destination.

In his book, *Let Your Life Speak*, Parker Palmer says, "Disabused of our illusions by much travel and travail, we awaken one day to find that the sacred center is here and now—in every moment of the journey, everywhere in the world around us, and deep within our own hearts."[3] The ability to live in the moment and recognize the beauty around us allows us to snatch up new adventures that help keep our vocation fresh and alive. There is something we can learn every day if we take the time to slow down and embrace the moment.

One of my constant battles is the transition from "doing" to "being." Most of my years have been spent doing something—schooling, graduating, Residency, mission work. What God is calling us to do is to be in a relationship with Him. He has done all of the hard work by dying on a cross to give us the opportunity to be in a relationship with Him. When we live in the moment, we are able to make our vocation and passion fluid and have the highest impact by constantly grabbing new journeys and adventures as they come our way. If we are too focused on the destination, these opportunities pass us by.

REDIRECTING

Early in their lives, I told my two nieces that I would take them anywhere in the world to do a service project at the end of their junior year of high school. My oldest niece, Sarah Hoffman, chose to go to Kenya to distribute soccer balls in orphanages, a special needs center, and underserved schools with my friend Robyn Moore. Sarah was familiar with my mission work and became interested in Africa at a very young age.

Prior to our trip to Kenya, she involved her soccer team and schoolmates in collecting equipment. By the time we left, we had plenty of soccer balls with a pump and patches to go with each one, in addition to numerous t-shirts from past soccer tournaments. Everywhere we went, she was kicking a soccer ball, which, more often than not, would start a game. She played every evening with boys who were mostly barefoot or wearing flip flops in the neighborhood where we stayed. Two brothers had one pair of shoes so each wore one shoe. At schools and orphanages, the children were always excited to put away whatever they had been using for a ball to try out a "real" soccer ball. Most of their soccer balls were plastic bags tied up with whatever they could find. Not only did Sarah play with the children, she also played with a Maasai tribe, as well as pick-up games with men on the beaches in Mombasa.

I loved watching how she was accepted in the games as though she had played with the Kenyans her entire life. Even though Sarah had seen pictures I

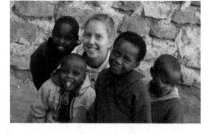

had taken from previous mission trips, physically being in an under-served area was eye-opening for her. She could immediately see the benefits of how she was helping the children.

My other niece, Amy Hoffman, chose to go to Central African Republic. I had recently made several trips to CAR, and she was interested in the work we were doing with community-based primary health care (CBPHC). Wanting to make an impact herself, she wasn't sure what kind of project she could do. I said, "Amy, there is so much you can do by helping in the clinic, meeting with the people in the village to continue the work with developing CBPHC, and playing with the children."

She responded, "Aunt Susan, I have no medical knowledge to do anything in the clinic and don't know about public health and education. And what good am I doing if I'm just playing with the children?" I said, "You're being an ambassador of good will, Amy, which will help in ways that you won't be able to see, but will be immensely impactful nonetheless."

Anne Goldsmith, a wonderful friend, joined us on our adventure. I met Anne when her husband was a fellow Resident with me. On our way to CAR, we stopped in Kenya to visit a couple of Robyn Moore's orphanages. Robyn had given us a list of items the children either needed or would enjoy. The list was a great starting point for Amy as she narrowed in on finding her value.

Once we arrived, she began measuring the impact she was making. The seemingly small acts of weighing babies, playing games, taking pictures and then showing the image to the children, who were seeing their image for the first time, were all large acts because the people she touched knew she cared about them. It also helped me immensely because, for the first time, I wasn't the blondest and whitest, so people flocked to her, which meant that I could have the chance to enjoy watching Amy interact with the Central African Republicans.

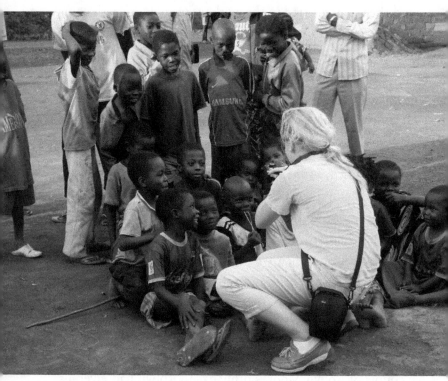

One night in particular was a highlight for Amy and Anne. On a Friday night around 9 p.m., as we were all in bed in the same room, we heard drumming and cheering coming from Gallo, the nearby village. We all looked at each other and then I noticed that Anne and Amy were having a conversation with their eyes. They both knew I needed my sleep and would not be getting out of bed. Amy's intrigue got the best of her as she left our room to inquire about the drumming. Anne then poked her head out of the room to hear the story. Ester, our host, said, "Every Friday night in the village is a time for fellowship, music, and dance." Being a teenager *and* a dancer, Amy's eyes lit up! When would an opportunity to see traditional African drumming and dance present itself again? Anne was hesitant, not wanting to get out of her pajamas; however, one look at the longing in Amy's eyes to follow the call of the drums was too much for Anne to resist. Amy was the first back to the bedroom, quickly changing into jeans. Anne followed, but first turned to me and said with resolution, "Amy gave me her 'look' and I could not resist." Anne remembers this part of the trip well:

> At the dance, our plan was to keep a low profile, not draw attention to ourselves, stand back and watch for a short time. We did not want to create attention or cause disruption to their festivities. After walking at least two miles, we headed into the bush, following the sound of the drums and singing. We stopped at the tree line, out of sight to absorb all that was upon us. Several small fires lit up the night. There were two circles of people. The first, a smaller group, was comprised of elderly villagers adorned in traditional headwear and skirts swirling in bursts of color, men in traditional long shirts, surrounded by men drumming on small and colorful traditional drums. Individuals took turns moving to the center of the circle, dancing, singing, and laughing. The second, a larger group of teenagers and young adults, was decked out in jeans and T-shirts. We knew this was their time to express themselves because we had never seen these clothes at any other time. Instead of drums, they were dancing to pop music from around the

world, playing on a battery-operated boom box. Amy's dance toes started to twitch.

We soon noticed our presence had been discovered. Even in the dark, it's hard for a white person to hide in Africa. A few looks and finger points came our way. As the number increased, community elders walked closer to keep a protective eye on us. We relaxed and appreciated the awe-inspiring evening that will forever be one of the most magical nights of my life. As Amy's dancing feet could no longer keep still, we moved to the circle of the young crowd, and Amy blended with the other kids. Through hand gestures and a weak attempt on my part at dancing in place, a young man figured out what I was saying. He invited Amy inside the circle to the dance floor. Amy jumped in with both feet. Standing in a crowd, I raised my camera and caught a picture of Amy in mid leap, the joy in her heart was evident by the smile on her face; she was beaming! To this day, I still can feel the joy we both enjoyed that night.

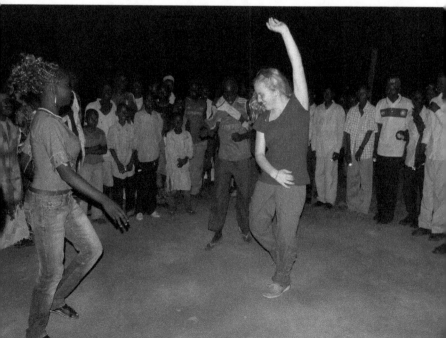

CONCEPT 4

Four years later, when asked how the trip to CAR changed the course of her life, Amy replied, "I saw firsthand the complexities and challenges of international aid. CAR also was not 'just another African country.' It's a country that has its own history and diversity of cultures. This first trip to CAR challenged me by revealing my naivety and forced me to confront it. The trip changed my life course because it showed me the intricacies of medicine and public health. Medicine especially requires cultural competency, compassion, and creativity. Community health is a powerful tool to educate individuals and bring a community together to set and achieve health goals. This trip piqued my interest in community health, especially within underserved communities."

One major difference between the experience of Sarah and Amy is that Sarah spent more time *doing* and Amy spent time *being*. Since their return, they have both been more aware of the needs of all people, here and away. Sarah is in graduate school for kinesiology and nutrition, monitoring physiologic factors of the women on the soccer team. Amy is taking a gap year as she applies to medical schools. During college, she did much to help vulnerable populations throughout Baltimore, her local community. She said her time in CAR enabled her to be more effective in helping the downtrodden and those most in need: "Before helping a low-income or underserved population, it is imperative to learn about their history and goals. If I can approach volunteering and helping others from a standpoint rooted in understanding, I am able to contribute much more."

My destination has changed so many times, I am not sure I even still have one. It is only recently that I have had the courage and strength to start making plans for the future. Like so many, my fear is that if I look ahead, something drastic will happen again, erasing my plans. Looking back on my life, I knew that the motor vehicle accident causing my TBI would—and has—changed my life drastically. Any destination I was thinking about was erased like a vapor, which is hard for people to understand since a head injury is not something seen outwardly by others; therefore, quickly forgotten by those not living with the trauma. The journey—and no longer the destination—became my life. My goal every morning is just to make it through another day. God calls us to be in a relationship with Him, which means He will take care of directing us to what He wants us to do. I know personally that that is so much easier said than done. One of the devotional books I am currently using is *Jesus Calling* by Sarah Young. During the course of writing this book, I realized that I had never read the devotion for March 24, the day of my accident. I don't know why I hadn't read it. It says:

> This is a time in your life when you must learn to let go: of loved ones, of possessions, of control. In order to let go of something that is precious to you, you need to rest in My Presence, where you are complete. Take time to bask in the Light of My Love. As you relax more and more, your grasping hand gradually opens up, releasing your prized possession into My care. You can feel secure, even in the midst of cataclysmic changes, through awareness of My continual Presence. The One who never leaves you is the same One who never changes: *I am the same yesterday, today, and forever.* As you release more and more

things into My care, remember that I never let go of your hand. Herein lies your security, which no one and no circumstance can take from you.[4]

Wow. I can honestly say that I would not change anything that has happened in my life, because it has brought me exactly to this place, writing this book. Are there days I wish I was the person I was before my TBI? Of course. It wasn't until 14 years later on Good Friday that I had a revelation about my accident that helped me move on: As I was driving to Minneapolis that day, strong winds made it hard for me to stay on the road, forcing me to keep both hands on the steering wheel at all times. As I passed a semi-truck, I felt the pull of the wind change and I gripped even harder to stay on the road. Even though I don't remember the accident that led to my TBI, I have been told what happened. Add to that, I was driving a rear-wheel drive van that was over-packed in the back. Carmen Keller, the passenger in the front seat, recalls there was no question it was an accident caused by the combination of circumstances. Fourteen years later, I had a revelation: I needed to forgive myself. Even though the accident was just that . . . an accident, I needed to take responsibility for the fact that I was driving, accident or not.

Second, I recognized that I had to look at my TBI in the same way I looked at my life in Africa and the United States, with a little twist. With my trips between Africa and the U.S., I had to immerse myself in the environment I was in at the moment. A similar view applies to my TBI. There are times when I find myself slipping back to wishing I had the thought process I had before my TBI when ultimately that is futile. It is what it is. When I think about how things were before my TBI, it does nothing to help my living in the moment.

God truly is in control. I wish I could remember that more than I do. I would handle changes much easier . . . unlike my reaction at Tenwek Hospital when I lost myself in a destination and forgot my real purpose. Here's the story: The Lindholm family and I had an opportunity to go on an overnight safari with a couple other missionaries. Even though I had only been working at the hospital for two weeks, I was ready for a break. When I think back on it, that fact alone is sad. My first week *had* started with that very long day I noted earlier. Okay, I'm done making excuses. The day of our safari was here. We were packed and ready to be picked up at 8 a.m. by a safari van. We waited and waited and waited for the van to arrive. There is a saying in Africa, TIA (This Is Africa), which often refers to time schedules. Communication between Nairobi and rural Kenya, which is where we were, was difficult at best. We finally received word that since we had not "confirmed" our trip, it was canceled.

Bad Reaction Number One: With my mind completely focused on two days off, we were expected to switch gears immediately and get back to work. My first response was, "I can't believe it! No one is expecting us at work!" Thankfully, this was all fuming inside so no one knew what I was feeling. I guess they do now. The reason we were needed at the hospital was because one doctor was home with chest pain and another became ill, so the only doctors available were surgeon Dr. Michael Johnson, Roger, and me. If we had gone on the safari, Dr. Johnson would have been left to run the entire hospital. However, I still had a bad attitude in my heart, which proved hard to conceal. As two events unfolded, my selfish attitude was quickly reversed.

First, a patient in surgery with an uncommon blood type needed blood. None was available. Fortunately, Roger's blood was a match and he was able to donate. Then, I was called to Labor and Delivery around 2 a.m. to help with a difficult delivery. I determined a Cesarean section was needed, called the surgeon, and waited so I could assist with the surgery. When Dr. Johnson arrived at the Operating Theatre, he told me to do the surgery and he would assist. What? Did I hear him correctly? I did! After assisting with many such surgeries, this was the first time I was lead surgeon. The first incision to the final closing stitch took less than an hour—not bad for a rookie. Even though it was 4:15 a.m. and we were leaving at 6:30 a.m. for another attempt at a safari, my heart was back where it needed to be, living moment by moment, trusting God to have the big picture.

Speaking of living moment by moment, I do realize that some moments are harder than others, which leads to Bad Reaction Number Two. Picture this moment in time.

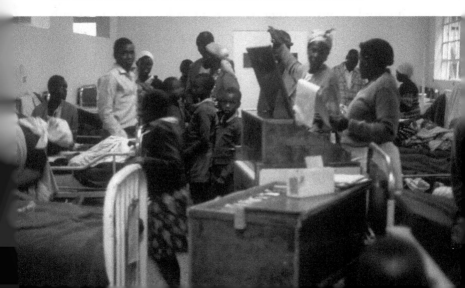

REDIRECTING

I had 58 patients in my 40 beds, and at one point in time I was trying to *simultaneously* manage a 28-year-old woman who was confused and psychotic with a blood sugar level of 607 (normal is around 100). Another patient was a 26-year-old woman, six months pregnant with malaria whose temperature spiked to 105 degrees F, with the fetal heart rate up to 180 beats per minute (too fast). Two other women picked that time to develop acute abdominal pain. Yet another patient, this time a 55-year-old woman who suddenly developed chest pain and shortness of breath, broke out in a sweat and then stopped breathing. She took priority, so resuscitative efforts were started but unsuccessful. She died. A patient started to hyperventilate with all the commotion, so I instructed one of the nurses to get a paper bag. She came back with a plastic bag and when I told her it had to be paper, she resigned and left crying. I was beside myself!

Every doctor working at Tenwek Hospital was given one day off a week. Mine was Tuesdays. This was the only full day that I could decide what to do with my time. One day, I went to a village with the Community Health Workers to help give immunizations; another day, I went to Kericho to help with grocery shopping for all the missionaries; many were spent writing, reading, and relaxing. On one particular Tuesday, Joan Lindholm and I walked to Silabwet, a neighboring village, to buy a serving bowl. We didn't have much time so we walked at a very brisk pace, and though I don't know the distance, we walked for over an hour. In no time, I was huffing and puffing and sweating. Upon returning home, I decided it was a good day to go to the hospital and take pictures, a nice leisurely activity, done at my own pace, and resting as needed. Silly me to think that there would be anything restful to do at the hospital.

Eventually, I went into the Operating Theatre where the surgeon was working on a woman who had a Cesarean section, which itself went well, but the patient wouldn't stop bleeding. Faith, the laboratory technician, came rushing into the room and said, "We're out of O positive blood!"

Immediately, without thinking, I said, "I think I'm O positive."

Faith grabbed me by the arm, pulled me out of the room, outside, across the hospital grounds, to the laboratory. We looked like quite a pair as Faith was in front, still holding my arm as I was trying to keep up with her. With my camera around my neck, which I was trying to hold to keep it from swinging back and forth, hitting Faith in the back and me in the chest. Upon arrival to the lab, Faith had me lie down on a flat table, set my arm down over the side, pulled my lower eyelid down to make sure it was red enough which meant my hemoglobin was okay, and started looking for a vein. I decided this was as good a time as any to say, "I *think* I'm O positive."

"How sure are you?" Faith replied.

"Quite sure," I said.

"Good enough."

She found a vein quickly, and we both watched the bag fill with blood. Since we had a couple of minutes to spare, I said, "So, Faith, how is your day?"

"Busy as usual. How about you?"

"I'm having a great day. It's my day off."

"I'm glad you're here. We needed you."

By then the bag was full, she pulled the needle out of my arm, slapped a bandage on, handed me the bag filled with my blood, and gave me a little push toward the door, which was my cue to bring the blood back to the operating theatre.

As soon as I walked through the doors, someone snatched the bag and hung it for immediate transfusion. For some reason, I was surprised at how warm my blood felt through the bag. Since I had started to feel a little lightheaded, I thought it best to head home. Where was the juice and crackers? What about reclining in a lounger for a while after giving blood? TIA. This Is Africa. Walking home, I was getting woozy and broke out in a sweat, which intensified as I remembered that I hadn't rehydrated after our walk to Silabwet. One look at me and Joan said, "You're as white as a ghost!" I laid down, filled her in on the patient needing blood, and watched as she quickly left for the hospital to donate more blood. As I was crawling to the refrigerator to get some water, I thought *this is not what I was expecting for today*. I was indeed living in the moment as it evolved minute by minute.

Recently, a friend reminded me of something I had told her years ago. She has found it to be true time and time again. I had said, "How do you make God laugh? Make a plan." Plans I have made throughout my life have often been shattered and scattered. Even still, some situations do require that we plan ahead. Before we can make a meal, we need to buy groceries. Meetings and social events need to be scheduled. In Minnesota, before the first snowfall, I always put my shovel by my back door so I can dig my dog and me out of my house after a blizzard. Such actions require looking into the future, and making a plan to prepare for inevitable or likely events.

Sometimes, being prepared can save a life, as it did for an eight-year-old boy whose name I don't even know. He and his mother impacted my life in many ways. They lived with about 120,000 other Rwandan civilians, mostly from the Hutu tribe, in a refugee camp in southern Rwanda. The Tutsis had taken control from the Hutus a few months previously in a bloody battle that involved unfathomable, heinous massacres as discussed earlier. One day, the Tutsi-controlled government of Rwanda decided to disband the camp and send everyone back to their homes—even though they had no idea if any homes were still standing.

Unbeknownst to the government-led RPA (Rwandan Patriotic Army) and the UN, hiding in the center of this refugee camp was a large group of Hutu militia who did not want the camp disrupted as it would expose their hiding place. They knew that if they were found, they would either be killed or sent to prison; so they told the people in the camp to not leave. When the RPA arrived to disband the camp, the people found themselves literally in the middle of a battle between the RPA, well-armed with guns, and the Hutu militia, armed with guns and machetes.

Chaos erupted. People tried to flee, but had nowhere to run. The RPA was firing bullets into the crowd to force them to scatter, and the Hutu militiamen were killing the civilians and RPA with bullets and machetes. About 30 UN workers who witnessed this slaughter were unable to do anything to help, as they were grossly outnumbered and were just trying to stay alive. The following day, the UN workers went in to assess the damage. They stopped counting the dead when they reached 4,000. Those who had survived fled the area, spreading across a country already saturated with homeless nomads.

The eight-year-old boy was one of the casualties of this bloody massacre. He was barely alive, breathing with great difficulty when found later by the UN. Shrapnel was imbedded in his chest, causing a pneumothorax (air around one of the lungs, causing it to collapse). Knowing he would surely die if left behind, members of the UN brought him to the hospital in Kigali. I met him on Monday morning while making rounds at that hospital.

When he was strong enough to talk, he relayed the last words he heard his mother speak. As chaos broke out in the camp, she said, "Son, remember what I have told you every day since we arrived in camp. If fighting starts, run with the crowd. It's time to run. Don't worry about me. I'll find you when the fighting stops." He wanted to stay with her, but she knew his best chance of survival was to stay in the middle of the crowd and keep running. She was prepared, and had a plan that ultimately saved the life of her son. In so doing, her son had the opportunity to continue living; no longer with a plan, but in the moment—one day at a time.

Snuggled next to the boy on his hospital bed was a severely malnourished four-year-old girl. She sheepishly looked at us while clinging to the arm of her bedmate. In the hospital, these two children had quickly become inseparable. Wherever one was, the other was close by. They were both alone in the world, not knowing if they had any living relatives left in Rwanda. At night, the two children were put in their separate hospital beds but soon were found cuddled together in one bed. In fact, this was a fairly common phenomenon. In our orphanage, it was not unusual to walk into a room and see eight children crammed onto one bed even though they were surrounded by seven empty beds.

These two unlikely friends gave each other a reason to wake up in the morning. They had no plans to make. The past was too atrocious to think about; the future looked hopeless; but they could live in the moment, appreciating each breath they took.

There have been times in my life when it feels like the world is crumbling around me and my pilot light is out within me. These are the times when I need to close my eyes and visualize the crowded bed surrounded by empty ones, and bask in the knowledge that I am loved by a Creator who promises to provide all I need. Sometimes all we have to hold onto is the comfort provided through human touch, which can be enough to help us make it through the dark nights as we await the morning light.

The ultimate example of living in the moment comes from Jesus. The Bible is an amazing book in so many ways. In Mark 5:21-43, Jesus was on the shore of "the other side" on the Sea of Galilea when Jairus, a leader of the synagogue, fell at Jesus' feet, "and begged Him repeatedly, 'My little daughter is at the point of death. Come and lay Your hands on her, so that she may be made well, and live.'" Jesus went with Jairus and on the way, as usual, He accumulated a huge crowd around Him. One of the people, who had been bleeding for 12 years, somehow managed to get close enough to touch the back of Jesus' cloak, "for she said, 'If I but touch His clothes, I will be made well.' Immediately her hemorrhage stopped; and she felt in her body that she was healed of her disease. Immediately aware that power had gone forth from Him, Jesus turned about in the crowd and said, 'Who touched my clothes?'" Imagine the reaction of the disciples and everyone else surrounding Jesus. They must have thought Jesus was crazy!

Think about a time when you were in the middle of a moving crowd, people bumping into you, everyone touching each other while jostling around. Now imagine stopping, turning around, and asking, "Who touched me?" As Jesus looked around the crowd, the woman, trembling with fear, came to Him and explained what happened. "He said to her, 'Daughter, your faith has made you well; go in peace, and be healed of your disease.'"

At the same time Jesus was talking to the woman, people had come to Jairus and told him his daughter had died, so not to bother bringing Jesus by the house. Jesus overheard them and said, "Do not fear, only believe." For Jairus, the parent who originally tracked down Jesus, that statement must have been difficult to embrace at that particular moment. His daughter had died while Jesus was taking His time looking for a woman who had touched Him!

Jesus allowed three of His disciples to accompany him to the home of Jairus where they found a huge commotion. People were weeping and wailing, going on and on, as though someone had died, which is what they believed. When Jesus entered the home and told them the girl was only sleeping, their wailing turned to laughter. They were actually laughing at Jesus for making such a ridiculous statement! He went into the child's room, told her to wake up, which of course she did immediately, and then started walking here and there. Jesus raising a child from the dead was the main focus.

Why am I making such a big deal out of this story? If you forget about the main story of Jesus raising a child from the dead, a great story indeed, there is another big story that can be missed. Imagine being Jairus, the father of a sick child who believed Jesus could make her well. I would be in a mad rush to get back home with Jesus to heal my child. And yet, Jesus takes His time and actually *stops* when He feels power moving through Him. Who wouldn't be furious that Jesus hadn't kept walking and maybe picked up His pace a bit? However, Jesus feels something within Himself, stops, heals a woman, and continues on to raise a child from the dead. He doesn't allow the opportunity to pass. He embraces the moment. Oh my goodness, I cringe when I think about how many times I pass up the moment.

REDIRECTING

I am driving
I am late for work
Spilling coffee down my whitest shirt
While I'm flossing and I'm changing lanes
Oh yeah

Now I'm driving
Through the parking lot
Doing eighty, what the heck why not
Watch it lady,
'Cause you're in my spot

I can't stand still
Can I get a witness
Can you hear me
Anybody, anybody
I think I'm running just to catch myself

I get on the ladder, I corporately climb
I wave at my life as it passes me by every day

When I meet God, I will have a question
I just forgot the question
I think I am running just to catch myself

—Mark Schultz, Running Just to Catch Myself

CONCEPT 5

Look North for Direction on Responsibility and Calling

Maybe it's a father working through the long night
Maybe it's a mother trying to raise her kids right
Maybe it's a prayer on a long drive home

Maybe it's a soldier fighting on the front line
Maybe it's a preacher laying down his own life
Maybe when You gave Your Son to die
That's what love looks like

—Among the Thirsty, *What Love Looks Like*

On August 10, 2016, NPR posted a story on the Internet entitled "Because I Can: Cyclist Kristin Armstrong Wins Third Gold Medal at Age 42," written by Bill Chappell. Kristin is the first cyclist ever, male or female, to win three gold medals in consecutive Olympics since 1896. One would think this fact alone means that all she does is train in cycling. Not so. As a world-class athlete, she sees the importance of maintaining balance in her life. She said, "Working at a great hospital in Boise, Idaho, and being a mom has been my secret weapon. It provides me balance, and it keeps me on track, and it keeps me super focused." She works as Director of Community Health at St. Luke's Hospital in Boise. "It's a dream job," she said. "I love it." This is a woman who is living her vocation, calling, and passion all while maintaining perspective on her responsibilities.

As is probably obvious, I am close to both my nieces. An example of my strong bond with Sarah occurred when she was young. She asked her mom, Kathy, "How do you know who you will marry?" Kathy responded, "You marry someone you love very much and want to spend your life with." Before she could say more, Sarah responded, "Well, that would be Aunt Susan!" When I was in Bosnia, Sarah was 5 years old. The only way I could communicate to people outside of the country was by fax.

One day, I received a fax from my sister Kathy saying, "I don't know what to do. Sarah is so worried about you that she is not functioning well. She hears all the bad news about Bosnia and can't stop worrying. I think you might have to come home." Wow! A conundrum indeed. I was confident that God had called me to Bosnia and the work we were doing was changing lives. I was the only doctor on our team which meant if I left, the medical team would consist of one person, nurse Tana. Don't get me wrong; Tana is fantastic, and if she left and I stayed, the result would be the same—one medical person. What was I to do? Did my responsibility for Sarah's well-being take precedence over my calling to Bosnia? At that time, faxes were a new thing and receiving one did not seem as real as getting a letter in the mail. Sarah said she would feel better if she got a letter from me.

I sent Kathy a fax for Sarah, telling her 1) I was safe; 2) I wasn't in the areas where fighting was occurring; 3) I had a map showing where the land mines were buried; and 4) there was nothing I wanted more than to come home safely and give her a big hug.

It was all true: 1) I was safe, compared to other areas; 2) fighting can be defined in a number of ways; 3) I had a map showing that we were working in the highest risk of land mines, but she did not need to know all the details; and 4) I really did want nothing more than to get home safely and give my nieces a big hug. Kathy folded the fax, put it in an envelope, addressed it to Sarah from me, and mailed it. Sarah felt better and I was able to stay in Bosnia. In the end, all was well. However, there was a period of a few days where I struggled between responsibility and calling.

One time when I was visiting Kathy, Mark, Sarah, and Amy, I had barely gotten out of my car before Amy came bounding out the front door, leaped into my arms, and gave me a huge hug. While bounding and leaping she said, "Aunt Susan, Aunt Susan! I have good news and bad news for you." We were at the hugging part when she finished her exclamation. I tilted my head back so I could look in her eyes as she continued, "The good news is that Sarah and I get to live with you!" Hmmm. I looked in the distance, searching my brain, trying to remember when Kathy and Mark asked me if I could take care of Sarah and Amy while they were away. Nothing came to mind. I looked back at Amy who now had a frown on her face as she said, "The bad news is that Mommy and Daddy have to die first." Ah hah, now I got it. Kathy and Mark must have told their daughters that if Mom and Dad died, they would live with me, and I would raise them.

The decision Kathy and Mark made was not done lightly and we discussed it thoroughly before they made it official. Their concern was a valid one. If I was guardian of Sarah and Amy, would I continue to do mission work in areas that put my life in imminent danger? If so, they were not comfortable giving me legal guardianship. Wow. It took only a couple of heart-beats before I knew what to say. "If I were guardian of Sarah and Amy, that would be my number one calling. I will not leave them without a parent." I think the reason my answer came so quickly is because God would not call me away from my work overseas unless He had a good reason. My nieces surely would be the reason.

There are times we all make choices that go against what our family, friends, and society think we ought to do, which puts us in a position to defend our decisions. Often the tension comes from the dichotomy of responsibility and calling. My choice to go back to Rwanda and cancel my trip to Peru was one of the hardest decisions for my family and friends. Cindy Bateman, my best friend during medical school, had invited me to join her on a trip to a remote area in Peru where we would be providing basic health care. But I had an unmistak-ably strong feeling that I needed to be in Rwanda. It was a feeling that plagued me. I contacted Cindy and canceled my trip to Peru. There were some who blatantly said they could not support me if I went back to a place that was so evil. They knew how difficult it was for me to be in Rwanda, and my well-being was front and center in their minds. All I could say was that I totally understood where they were coming from, but they were seeing the situation from a totally different angle than I was. I knew that God had clearly called me to be a light in the darkness, adding my light to the light of other Christians called to do the same.

At times, it is hard to discern between what God is trying to tell me and what I *want* God to tell me. Going back to Rwanda was a decision I made based on knowing that God was calling me to that place of darkness for His purposes. I was intentionally listening to God on the deepest level. It's hard to explain in words.

On the other hand, there are times when I look at signs as being truth when there is no special meaning intended. When I suffered the knee injury I mentioned earlier, my life started to unravel. For self-preservation and because I felt I lost my sense of purpose, I became self-absorbed. For me, when I feel like I lack purpose, I either end up in the wilderness or I do something idiotic and impulsive, thinking it will give me purpose. The impulsive part I can partly blame on the head injury; the idiotic part is all on me.

Several months ago, for instance, I was a runner—someone who does whatever needs to be done—for Jeremy Camp and his band during a concert in Fargo, North Dakota. As I was talking with a few band members, I mentioned that I wanted to learn how to play the drums. They encouraged me to do it. "Do you have a drum set?" they asked. "No," I responded. Without any prodding on my part, Toby, the lead back-up singer and guitarist, looked on Craigslist and found a great deal on a used set, which happened to be in a town close to mine. We showed it to Leif, the drummer, who agreed it was a great deal. So I bought it. Had I ever even played a drum set? No, I played brass and piano. Had I ever considered the truth that I have difficulties multi-tasking and that it may be hard to have all four extremities doing something different at the same time? That thought eluded me. So why did I want to play the drum set?

When I took a moment to think through this question, I realized it was because I like to listen to someone play the drums, and they look cool as their whole body gets into the beat of the song. It would have been helpful to have made that distinction before buying an entire set of drums. At the time, I justified it by saying, "Everything's falling into place, so it must be the right thing to do!" However, I failed to ask the right questions. What is my life telling me? Will this fit into my vocation? Do I have the spare money? What is the responsible thing to do? I did not listen before I leapt.

Responsibility in relation to our calling takes on many forms. One area I struggle with is the responsibility of taking care of me while serving others, especially in Africa. Many of us in caregiver roles have an easier time taking care of the needs of others but at the expense of our own. To care for ourselves feels selfish. Parker Palmer, author of *Let Your Life Speak: Listening for the Voice of Vocation,* puts this dilemma in a healthy, true perspective, " . . . self-care is never a selfish act—it is simply good stewardship of the only gift I have, the gift I was put on earth to offer to others. Anytime we can listen to true self and give it the care it requires, we do so not only for ourselves but for the many others whose lives we touch."[5] I love how this is worded. God created us to be who we are, for His purpose, and if we do not take care of the gift of life He has given us, we do not honor Him.

While in Southern Sudan, I struggled with the notion that I had enough food while the Sudanese I was helping did not. We, as Ex-Patriots (non-Sudanese), had food flown in, and even though our food supply could sometimes get low, I always knew that I would not die of starvation, a valid concern for the people I was trying to help. I realized that even though we were living amongst the Sudanese by living in their village, we were still living in a bubble. And, even though we weren't eating extravagant meals, we still had food. We as caregivers knew we had to eat to remain healthy so that we could help others. Even Jesus needed to take care of Himself. There came a point when He needed to take a break and replenish His spiritual strength. Mark 1:35 reminds us, "In the morning, while it was still very dark, He got up and went out to a deserted place, and there He prayed."

My friend, Amy, and I recently discussed how she is able to balance her responsibilities with her callings. The reason I chose to interview Amy on this subject is because she manages to shuffle her two children, husband, job, vocation, hobbies, friends, and daily chores like no one else I know. She gives me a great perspective on what calling really is and can be. She shared with me the quote from Frederick Buechner, "The place God calls you to is the place where your deep gladness and the world's deep hunger meet." Sound familiar? I shared it in Concept 2 and asked you to stop and read it again.

Amy says that our calling is often seen as something big we do, something we are led to, and many times seen through the filter of a job. Remember, though, character and values flow out of who we *are* rather than what we *do*. When character and values work together and are in alignment, there is deep gladness, and we are equipped to meet the world's deep hunger. Amy believes that the root of the "world's deep hunger" is *being*; to be heard, to experience, to be kind, to give grace. It is quite possible that calling, at its core, is a whole lot simpler than we make it. Saint Mother Teresa captured this concept well when she simply said, "Do small things with great love."

Amy further explains, "I would say I have a calling to authenticity and alignment. I'm constantly making sure that what I am saying, doing, and believing are in alignment. I feel called to Kindness, Alignment, Truth, Grace. It's not a *doing* activity, rather who I am *being*. Responsibility is something that falls in the category of doing. I am responsible to complete tasks, meet deadlines, and care for people. I do these things with kindness, alignment, truth, and grace . . . that's who I strive to be. Daily, there is a pre-determined hierarchy of responsibilities that is part of how I go through life. My husband and my kids are first on that list. There are a lot of 'should' pressures and I have learned, mostly by failing many times, to be alert to the 'should' pressure and exchange it for things I really value—to be clear about what I have decided is important in my life. One thing I have become clear about is the importance of margins, meaning downtime. My family needs margins. My kids do best when they have lots of unscheduled time to play and just *be*. Whatever we do is filtered through the lens of 'do we have enough margins?' I have taken the perspective of saying *no* to the good, and saying *yes* to the best. It's a principle that can apply to all areas of life." Somehow, Amy lives this out beautifully.

Parents have the incredible responsibility of caring for their children and doing what they feel is in the child's best interest . . . indeed, it is their calling. The decisions we make in the United States are often completely different than those facing parents in other countries. One day, while working in our clinic in Southern Sudan, a mother came with her two children. One child, about three years old, was skin and bones, curled up in a basket meant for an infant.

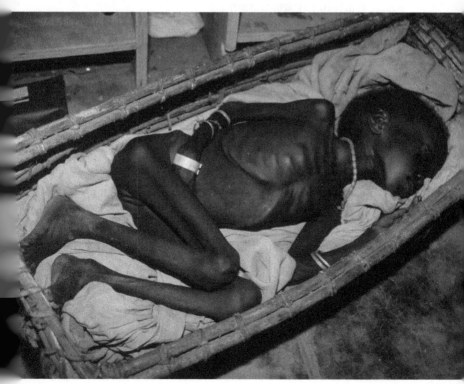

The mother appeared very detached and did not lift the child out of the basket or even look in her direction. Since the child was severely dehydrated, we started giving IP (intra peritoneal) fluids. Basically, we stuck a needle into the abdominal cavity to deliver fluids rather than the intravenous method (IV). This delivery system is a way to give a larger amount of fluid over a shorter time period as the fluid in the abdomen is slowly absorbed. In the meantime, the mother was giving her full attention to the 6-month-old, well-nourished sibling. I couldn't believe my eyes! In my journal I wrote, "I'm sure the mother had given up on the older child a few months ago, but finally brought her to the clinic when she wouldn't die." I was speaking out of anger, praying there wasn't truth in my frustration.

Four months earlier, the mother had brought her daughter to the feeding center in our village; however, the child became ill within a few days. The mother left the village with her daughter to find traditional medicines and treatment, assuring the staff she would be back when the child was better. She did not return to Ulang village until this day when we met at the clinic for the first time. It was so hard to watch the mother be so *detached* to one child and so *attached* to another. I did not understand!

She agreed to stay at the clinic so we could give her sick child fluids and food. We gave the mother a cup of water and showed her how to give her daughter a spoonful at a time. Sometimes when we looked in her direction, she was drinking the water herself or giving it to her younger child. What? How can she do that when her older daughter so desperately needs it? After a few days without seeing the family in the clinic, I became concerned. Upon inquiry, I discovered they were going to the feeding center, which was encouraging, but the older girl died the next day.

At the time, it was difficult to wrap my head around what this mother did to her daughter. In the United States, she would have been turned over to Social Services. Ah hah. Therein lies my problem. I was thinking with my American brain when I needed to be fully immersed in Southern Sudan and trying to see from their eyes. We cannot even begin to fathom the decision this mother had to make. She could use her limited resources to try to keep both children alive with the real risk of both dying. Or she could choose one child to focus her resources on to make sure she could at least save one child.

Later, I learned that this is a common phenomenon in countries that lack the resources needed to feed everyone. We truly cannot know what we would do if in her place. Once I looked at her situation through her eyes, I knew instantly I was in no position to judge.

Give me Your eyes for just one second
Give me Your eyes so I can see,
Everything that I keep missing,
Give me Your love for humanity.

Give me Your arms for the broken-hearted
The ones that are far beyond my reach.
Give me Your heart for the ones forgotten.
Give me Your eyes so I can see.

—Brandon Heath, *Give Me Your Eyes*

One of the most thought-provoking movies I have seen is *At Play in the Fields of the Lord,*[6] which is described as, "An adventure beyond the limits of civilization, faith, and passion." The movie chronicles three different approaches, through three different character types, to interacting with the Niaruna tribe in the Brazilian Amazon River basin. Two approaches are Christian-based and the other, humanitarian-based. One Christian-based approach was shown in a missionary couple who lived apart from the tribe and was there to convert the tribe to Christianity by word alone—no actions and no relationship building. The humanitarian-based approach was extreme and depicted through a mercenary who flew his plane over a Niaruna village, parachuted out of the plane before it hit a mountainside, and then stripped naked on his way to the village, ready to become *one of them*. The other Christian-based approach, and last to enter the scene, were Christian missionaries who, with their young son, came to live among the Niaruna, preaching the Gospel while trying to understand the natives, helping them when possible. Initially, this was the family I could most relate to after working with those in need. My approach had been to spend time learning the culture and building relationships with the Nationals before teaching anything. I also tried to avoid preaching.

The movie takes a twist, which forces the audience to question all three approaches. The first couple, living among other expatriates (foreigners), did not know what the people really needed besides the truth of the Gospel. The other Christian family was devastated when their son died from black water fever, a severe complication of malaria. His father continued their work, while the mother literally became insane from grief. She needed help desperately, and wasn't getting what she wanted from her husband—a one-way ticket home. Her husband decided to stay despite his wife roaming naked in the jungle, speaking nonsense, and making a fool of herself, her family, and her religion. While this part of the story was transpiring, the mercenary found the wife of the first missionary couple, bathing in the river. They shared a kiss of death. The bathing wife had the common cold, and while they both had immunity—the Nationals did not. The mercenary brought the virus back to his village and watched all of them, one by one—including his Niaruna wife—die of a virus their bodies had not seen before.

The tension between calling and responsibility was portrayed best by the couple whose son had died. The father was so set on staying to help the Niaruna that he lost sight of the needs of his wife. No one but he knows what was in his heart and what was driving him to make decisions, but it does cause one to ponder what the right decision might be. Only he knows how he was listening to God.

The first time I watched the movie I recognized that, despite good intentions, we can do immense harm when reaching out to the world. The burden of responsibility for what I was doing became very real, and I became much more intentional about building relationships and learning from the local people before anything else.

Sometimes, though, our responsibilities are in conflict with our personal ethics. My first day working in Southern Sudan as the only physician in the village, hit me like a ton of bricks. Forever etched in my mind are the faces of a mother and her son, who appeared to be between nine to 12 months old, who came to the clinic for care. He was my second patient of my first day. One look at the child caused my stomach to somehow find its way to my throat. He was very sick. Putting my hand on his abdomen immediately let me know he had a high fever, and he was taking breaths way too fast for his little body. I could tell his heart was getting tired because of his weak pulse. My diagnostic conclusion was that he was dehydrated and septic, meaning infection had found a way into his blood stream, carrying bacteria to every part of his body. Where the infection started will remain a mystery.

Herein lies the ethical dilemma that made it difficult for me to determine my responsibility. Medically, the only chance this boy had for survival was an injection of an antibiotic into his vein. However, deep in my heart, I was sure he would die even if given the antibiotic since he appeared so close to death already. However, without the injection, he had no chance at all to survive. However, however. Why was this a dilemma? Because we had a very limited supply of injectable antibiotics. Do I use some on this child who would most likely die anyway, knowing this was his only chance at surviving? Do I save it for a child who needs injectable antibiotics and has a better chance of living? How would I feel if I used it, the child dies, we ultimately run out of IV antibiotics, and a child comes to the clinic that would have lived, but died because we didn't have the antibiotics? All of these questions were racing through my brain at lightning speed. I opted to give the IV antibiotics. He died 30 minutes later, the first death to occur at the clinic. The fact that it happened five minutes after I started work did not help improve my self-confidence. His mother cried very softly, gently laid her son back in his basket, and left for her long walk back to her village. She initially had left her village in the morning of the previous day and arrived in Ulang in the evening. Patiently she waited through the night for the clinic to open. Now she had another full day of walking, this time carrying her dead son, with the added weight of grief. If only she lived closer, her son would have survived. If only he was seen as soon as they arrived in the village. If only, if only. But I still questioned. Was I irresponsible? Did I make the wrong decision? I had to remind myself that the outcome of an event does not change whether the original decision was right or wrong. Outcomes are in God's hands. I made the best decision I could at the time and that was all I could do.

I believe our responsibility to our calling is to listen to God *continually*—at this moment in time, under the circumstances at present—and do our best at following His lead. Maybe He's telling us to get up and move. Maybe He's saying stay put. It doesn't matter if you are a janitor at a business or the CEO, a cook at a fast food joint or the fanciest restaurant in town, we are all equal in God's eyes. Our responsibility is to be *our* best at whatever we are being called to do, not *the* best. Not only what we are called to *do*, also who we are called to *be*.

The ultimate responsibility—the calling for each of us—is to *love*. Love ourselves, our neighbors, the loveable, the unlovable, our enemies, those close and far away, even the worst criminals. In Matthew 5:43, Jesus says, "Love your enemies and pray for those who persecute you." It is hard for me to continue to despise someone when I pray for them. While it does take perseverance and time, gradually the hate turns to love. Saint Stephen, the first Christian martyr, was able to show love to his enemies immediately. When he was being stoned to death for preaching the truth, he said, "'Lord, do not hold this sin against them.' When he had said this, he died," (Acts 7:60) This sounds a bit like Jesus on the cross. He loved until the end, and continues to do so today. We are called to do the same.

Friday, came home, waved to a neighbor I don't know
He smiled at me and I believed he was doing just fine
His eyes can't lie
There's something tearing him up on the inside
I wonder what it is, I should ask him
But I've got my own life
Will I pass by?
Or am I gonna take the time?

This is what we're here for
To show the world how You love it
This is what we're made for
To lay it all down like You did
When we feel useless, You still use us
Help us not forget
This is what we're here for

—The Afters, *What We're Here For*

CONCEPT 6

The Power of One Ripples in All Directions

It all begins with one, the power of one
Joining the hundreds of millions of people believing

In one, the power of one

Don't hang around
Stand up or sit down and believe
We can change the world together

We can change the world together

—Israel Houghton, *The Power of One*
(*Change the World*)

In 1994, I saw the movie *The Power of One*,[7] and it has topped my list of favorites ever since. The movie takes place in South Africa during apartheid (an Afrikaans word that means a state of being apart, or "aparthood"), spanning WWII. The story follows the life of an English boy, PK, from birth into early adulthood. Being the only English boy in an Afrikaner school, PK learns what it is like to be persecuted. Afrikaners are white South Africans originally descended from the Dutch. When PK's mother dies, he becomes an orphan and is sent to live with his grandfather. He meets Doc, a German pianist, who takes him under his wing, teaching PK how to think for himself. Doc said that school will teach him the facts, but original thought comes from nature. "Africa is my classroom," stated Doc to PK on one of their nature walks. "Any question you ever have, the answer you'll find in nature if you know where to look and how to ask; and then you will have for yourself all of the brains you'll ever need."

At the start of WWII, Doc, being German, is imprisoned. PK visits him daily and soon meets Geel Piet, a black African prisoner, who teaches PK how to box. Geel Piet's motto for PK, "Little beat big when little smart. First with the head, then with the heart," went beyond the boxing ring. The prisoners are black Africans, many speaking only their native tribal language; PK learns how to speak them all. Amongst the prisoners, Geel Piet spreads the myth of the Rainmaker, one who unites all the tribes, and the tribes spread the word that PK may be the Rainmaker.

PK's next stop in life is the Prince of Wales, a school in Johannesburg where he continues to box, training in a multiracial gym. He meets Gideon Duma, a prominent boxer in Alexandra who is passionately fighting against apartheid. The minority white Afrikaners had control of the country and wanted to keep the black Africans suppressed with minimal to no rights. Duma challenges underdog PK to a boxing fight in Alexandra. If PK were to win, Duma would continue the myth that PK was the Rainmaker. If Duma won, the myth would falter.

PK wins in dramatic style and becomes an ally with Duma to stop apartheid. Duma tries to convince PK that they should work together to fight apartheid by teaching English to the black Africans: "We offer a good tomorrow in South Africa, but if we don't learn [English] and prove ourselves as equals, that hope will disappear. Disappear! And my people will grow tired, with tired will grow anger, with anger—violence."

As PK is trying to decide what to do, he remembers what Doc said to him as a child about how all answers can be found in nature. Therefore, PK returns to nature, looking for an answer. As he comes upon a waterfall, he stops and gradually hones in on the water until he can see individual drops of water. He had his answer. PK asks a professor if they could use a building on campus as a schoolroom. His professor says, "It's only about a dozen people you're talking about teaching, and how much difference will that really make?" PK responds, "A waterfall begins with only one drop of water, Sir, look what comes from that."

The first time I saw the movie, PK's response jumped right out of his mouth and into my heart, the biggest reason it has stayed number one on my movie list. At the end of the movie, the following quote lingers on the screen: "In South Africa and around the world, the struggle to gain human dignity and equal rights for all people continues. Changes can come from the power of many, but only when the many come together to form that which is invincible . . . the power of one."

It's true. The power of one can refer to an individual person who brings many together to work in community as one, with one goal, one purpose, one calling, one passion. Like PK. The power of one also can be looked at from the angle of one person who needs help and all the individual people needed to provide the help. One person can break the chain by not doing their part and stop the process completely, which means the person in need remains helpless. These real-life examples communicate each type of example.

First, we will look at the ripple effect of one person who is following his vocation, calling, and passion, and see where the ripples take us. Pediatric cardiologist and Pastor Dr. Kirk Milhoan continually shows how much good can come from the work of one person. The ripples from his work can be felt around the world. He and his wife, anesthesiologist Dr. Kim Milhoan, started a non-profit organization called For Hearts and Souls, which helps fund some of their work overseas.

Kirk, Kim, and I first met in October 2000 at a Christian conference. They were living in San Antonio, Texas; Kirk, working as a pediatric cardiologist, and Kim, finishing her Residency in Anesthesiology. At the time, I was working with a children's heart program. Our connection at the conference was God-ordained. I needed the help of a pediatric cardiologist and they needed a mission. Kirk, Kim, and I felt the collision of our deep gladness meeting the world's deep hunger. For Kirk, his flame changed the entire country of Mongolia.

Shortly before meeting Kirk, I was working with Dr. Byambasuren (Dr. B), the pediatric cardiologist in Mongolia, helping her choose children that were appropriate candidates for surgery in the United States. Being the only pediatric cardiologist in Mongolia, a country with a mortality rate of greater than 50 percent for anyone receiving simple heart surgery, she had a difficult job. In other words, surgery in her country was not an option for children with heart defects who weighed less than 50 pounds or whose cases were, in any way, complicated. Without surgery, these children inevitably would die from heart complications. Even with only a simple defect to fix, a child still had less than a 50 percent chance of surviving surgery.

Part of the reason for the high mortality was lack of education and lack of adequate equipment. The Mongolian surgeons did not have cardiac bypass machines that take over the function of the heart during surgery while the heart is stopped. Instead, they put the patient on a bed of ice, causing hypothermia (severe cold), which slows or stops the heart. When the surgery was completed, the patient was taken off the ice bed and warmed to normal temperature. It was a risky tactic that many people—young or old—simply couldn't survive.

Through our children's heart program, we were able to help some of the children by bringing them to the United States for the surgery they needed. However, in the long run, this was helping a select few and causing a dependency on the United States, which is not optimal for the long haul. I do not want to minimize the changes that were being made in the families and communities of those that were able to have surgery. At the time, it was their only hope of survival. What I am saying is that I did not have the expertise or the amazing abilities of Dr. Milhoan to constantly think outside the box and diplomatically deal with people at many levels of the government, the medical community, and other non-profit organizations. Kim helped with transports and used her anesthesiology skills during cardiac surgery. The Milhoan's housed many children, mothers, and translators in San Antonia when surgery was not possible in Mongolia.

Like manna from heaven, and only two months after our meeting, Kirk shared his expertise with Dr. B in Mongolia as I introduced Dr. B to Dr. Milhoan. The single flame of one determined man changed all of Mongolia forever.

Kirk spent time with Dr. B, educating her on how to effectively use an echocardiogram machine (ultrasound that looks at the function of the heart), which arrived from the United States a month before Kirk's arrival. Then, in 2003, Kirk brought his first medical team to screen all children for heart defects in the Aimags Province of Darkhan. The team listened to the hearts of the children in the district, and anyone with a heart murmur (suggesting a heart defect) was tested with a portable echocardiogram machine. Those children with imminent problems were sent to the U.S. through the children's heart program. By 2012, Kirk and his team had screened the children in every province in Mongolia!

Now that children who needed surgery were being identified, Kirk decided it was time to bring a surgical team from San Antonio to Mongolia. On their first surgical mission in 2005, their surgical equipment did not make it to Mongolia; time to think outside the box and figure out how to use what was available. The hospital in Mongolia had two old heart bypass machines that did not have all the required parts. They improvised by using a pickle jar for suction, and veterinarians gave them the suture they needed.

As they performed surgeries, they taught the Mongolian surgeons how to improve their surgical skills. In 2006, Kirk and other cardiologists started training the Mongolian doctors on how to perform heart catheterizations. Later, after Hurricane Katrina hit and while Kirk was stationed in San Antonio, he was given millions of dollars' worth of catheterization lab supplies by hospitals in the path of the hurricane, which he brought to Mongolia. Not only did this help with the pediatric cardiac catheterization efforts, it also built up the adult program so they could start treating coronary artery disease without surgery.

In addition to working in conjunction with the Mongolia Ministry of Health, Kirk also reached out to other non-government organizations, including a group from Korea, and shared resources that allowed other countries to become more involved. Once the heart surgery program was showing success, the Mongolian Hospital was able to get grants to help build up the Intensive Care Units and equip all of the Operating Rooms. In 2006, Kirk raised $50,000 to purchase 50 bypass circuits (equipment needed for heart surgery) and told the surgeons in Mongolia that he would give it all to them if they promised to stop performing heart surgery using the often-unsuccessful ice method.

What most missionaries want is to work themselves out of being needed. Dr. Kirk Milhoan did just that. Since 2000, Kirk has made 45 trips to Mongolia. There are now seven pediatric cardiologists trained by Kirk. The survival rate for patients who have had surgery done by the United States team was 96 percent. Now the survival rate for patients who have surgery done by Mongolian doctors is 95 percent.

The power of one. Of course, Kirk could not have accomplished this on his own, but through his own determination, he was able to produce a worldwide effort. Kirk said, "I come with fish and loaves of bread to God and don't tell Him what to do with it. I follow His lead." Dr. Milhoan was one drop of water that started a waterfall.

Let's take a look at this through the opposite lens. One that magnifies the effects of Kirk's work on the life of one of the heart-sick children. If any one person had neglected to do his or her part—thus breaking the chain of events—the life of this sick child, and others, would have been in jeopardy.

In 2001, Batchimeg was a 15-year-old girl dying of heart failure in Mongolia. I was in the process of arranging for two adolescents from Mongolia to go to Fargo, North Dakota, for heart surgery. One was Munkhbayar, a 16-year-old boy with the same diagnosis as Batchimeg, but his heart damage was not at an advanced stage. The second was a girl who was unable to make the trip after I discovered her mother was in the U.S. illegally and was unwilling to return to Mongolia, which is the only way we could get a visa for her daughter.

At the same time, I was in process of making plans for these two adolescents, I received a call from Dr. Kirk Milhoan who was in Mongolia on one of his heart defect screening missions. He said, "Susan, I am seeing a girl named Batchimeg who will die if she does not have surgery soon. Can we get her to the States?" I replied, "I'll work it out." I had worked with Kirk long enough to know that he did not mince words. I knew I needed to act fast. Maybe she could come to Fargo with Munkhbayar and take the place of the girl who couldn't go?

God had put all of this in motion before we were aware. In 2000, while visiting family in Fargo, I read a newspaper article in the *Fargo Forum* spotlighting the top women to watch that year. Highlighted on the list was cardiothoracic surgeon Dr. Roxanne Newman. I visited her to ask the obvious question, "Are you willing to perform surgery on two adolescents from Mongolia? For free?" Her immediate answer, "Of course!"

We had already identified Munkhbayar and the other female teenager who needed heart surgery and were waiting for the right situation to present itself. Now we had it! I sent Dr. Newman the videotapes of the two patients' echocardiogram, and she said both would be relatively simple cases. When I returned to her and said, "We have a bit of a situation on our hands. The echocardiogram of the girl you saw cannot come to the U.S. Are you willing to take someone else who is very sick, needs valve replacement, but doesn't have an echocardiogram?" Her response was God breathed, "I'll take care of whoever you bring me." Neither of us had a clue what we were up against.

The first hurdle cleared, I headed to the second hurdle—convincing the CEO of MeritCare Medical Center (now Sanford Medical Center) to waive all hospital expenses. In my experience, if I had the approval of the surgeon, the CEO was more likely to agree to help. Unfortunately, in this case, the CEO said, "No. We only provide charitable care for local people." A conundrum. Now what? As it turns out, I didn't have to do anything! Anesthesiologist Dr. Bob Brunsvold stepped up to the plate. He had heard about the two Mongolian children and was excited to do his part in their care. When Bob heard about the CEO's response, he immediately stormed into the

CEO's office and said, "How am I supposed to face my pastors when I have the opportunity to help save the lives of two people but cannot because the CEO of my hospital won't agree to provide the services for free?" By the time he left the CEO's office, we had the approvals we needed. Hallelujah!

Immediately, though, we faced another hurdle. We had to find a host church in Fargo who would provide support for the Mongolia group. At the time, my Dad was one of the pastors of First Lutheran Church, which is across the street from the hospital. Some of its congregants included Dr. Newman and Dr. Brunsvold. Asking the church to get involved and getting their approval was as easy as eating pizza. The church identified someone to coordinate and another to open her home to complete strangers, agreeing to care for them for six weeks. With Fargo now ready, it was time to focus on getting the Mongolians to North Dakota. The clock was ticking for Batchimeg, as her heart did its best to keep up with the strain of her damaged valve.

My friend, Kevin Wallevand, accompanied me to Mongolia with the intention of making a documentary. (*Flight for Life*, the documentary, was an Emmy award runner-up.) The time had come for us to fly to Ulan Bator, the capital of Mongolia. Or so we thought. Alas, when we arrived in Beijing, China, on a layover, we discovered our flight to Mongolia had been canceled, and was not to be rescheduled for three days. Three days! That was unacceptable. Batchimeg was literally living one day at a time!

We knew there was a plane flying out the next day, but were told there were no seats available. We needed to be on that plane! With Kevin's moral support, I asked to talk with the highest-ranking person because a girl's life depended on us getting to Ulan Bator the next day. "If we have to wait three days," I said, "you will have to reschedule a group of seven people, one of whom is dying, flying from Ulan Bator to Fargo, North Dakota, USA, with multiple plane changes." That got his attention. He didn't need to find a supervisor. He clicked some buttons and said he was able to get us the last two seats on the flight that left the next day. Yes! We both were determined to get there, even if it meant duct taping ourselves to the wings. Thankfully, that was not necessary.

When I walked into the Mongolian Hospital and saw Batchimeg for the first time, her smile consumed the room. She was sitting on the hospital bed, undernourished, next to her father whose face was etched with concern. I sat down, held her hand, gave her a smile of my own, and introduced myself with Dr. B translating. Even though Dr. Milhoan had warned me that she was very sick, I wasn't prepared for what I saw. I could actually see her heartbeats as they pulsed against her shirt at a fast rate.

After examining her, my mind was racing as I thought, "How will this girl ever make the flight halfway around the world from Mongolia to North Dakota?" Once my initial fear abated, I relied on the prayer that surrounded Kirk's decision to send her to the United States. Just as Kirk previously surmised, Batchimeg glowed with her smile and spirit, and I was immediately on board with him to get her to the States as soon as possible. I prayed, "Here I am, Lord. Use me. I need a miracle. I need your strength. I need you to take control of everything because I am inadequate on my own."

Batchimeg's father, with pain chiseled in his face, asked Dr. B a question and then both looked at me. Dr. B translated, "He wants to know if there is a chance that his daughter may die in your country." There was a moment of silence as he looked down at his fidgeting hands. I replied, "We have many, many people who are working hard, doing our absolute best, and will continue to do whatever is needed to bring Batchimeg back home, feeling better than she has in a very long time. I must be honest, your daughter is sick, and there is the possibility that she will not survive the surgery. You are being a very brave father by letting her go so far away to get treatment that is her only chance of surviving. I promise you that I have found the best surgeon in our country to do her surgery." All he could do was nod while fighting back tears. All I could do was pray.

Our departure at the airport was a mix of anticipation and sadness. Watching Batchimeg say goodbye to her father was gut-wrenching. As I wheeled her down the jet way, the last to get on the plane, we were immediately stopped by the flight attendant. As she watched Batchimeg's shirt move to the beat of her heart, she said, "There's no way this girl can get on the plane. She won't survive the flight. Look at her!" We both looked at her as she flashed us her beautiful smile. I looked back at the flight attendant who was momentarily mesmerized. That would be the flight attendant's weakness—Batchimeg's smile. "She will die for sure if she stays in Mongolia," I said. "Her only chance of survival is surgery in the U.S. I'm a doctor and take full responsibility for her, and I promise you that she won't die on this flight." There it was;

I said it and couldn't take it back. Lord, I need you now more than ever. Give me wisdom.

The flight attendant said, "Where are you sitting?" I handed her our boarding passes as Kevin helped the rest of the group find their seats. She looked at our seat assignments, then back to me, and one last look at Batchimeg before she looked back at me and said, "There are two empty seats in business class. You two will sit there so you can make her as comfortable as possible." I hadn't realized I had stopped breathing until she finished talking, and I took in a deep breath of air. Spontaneously, I gave the flight attendant a hug and said, "You are part of a chain of people who will save the life of this girl."

We arrived at Hector International Airport in Fargo, North Dakota, to a reception of many people, holding signs, smiling, waiting to embrace these strangers who immediately became friends. Batchimeg, her Aunt Bayanaa, and translator Oyunaa and I went directly to the hospital while Munkhbayar and his mom left to settle in with their host family.

Pediatric cardiologist Dr. Rod Rios was waiting for us at the hospital to do an echocardiogram. One look at Batchimeg and he was amazed she tolerated the long trip and absolutely astonished that she was still alive! Her left atrium, one of the four chambers of the heart, was three times larger than normal and her left ventricle (another chamber) was also large due to the diseased mitral valve. "I have never seen a heart this big," said Dr. Rios. "This is a very severely affected heart."

Dr. Rios consulted with Dr. Newman, the surgeon, and both agreed that the stakes were higher than anticipated and the surgery would be extremely high risk. Her father needed to be part of the decision-making; it was more likely that Batchimeg would die during surgery than live. Imagine the emotions of her father, receiving a phone call, months after his wife died, again being asked for permission to perform surgery on his daughter; now being told there was little chance she would make it through surgery alive. Knowing she would die without the surgery, he agreed to proceed.

Surgery was scheduled to occur two days later. Ione and Hillie, prayer warriors from First Lutheran Church, led the prayer team, covering every hour starting before surgery and continuing for 24 hours. There was so much behind-the-scenes work that was done by the church and others. Dr. Roxanne Newman opted to first operate on Munkhbayar to fix his valve, which was not as damaged, and his heart was in better condition.

As Dr. Newman was scrubbing in for surgery, she said, "For so long, we've gotten information, exchanged emails, and now we finally have a patient. It's totally different!" Munkhbayar's surgery went as planned and was finished in a couple of hours. When I went to the room where everyone was waiting, to give them the good news, his mother gave me the biggest, longest hug as she was shaking with relief. Every time I tried to step back, she pulled me in tighter. Best hug ever.

It was Batchimeg's turn at last. When her Aunt Bayanaa bent over the side rail on the stretcher to give Batchimeg one last kiss, she was so strong. As soon as Batchimeg went through the door into the surgical area, Bayanaa broke down. It's hard to fathom what was going through her mind, knowing there was greater than a 50 percent chance she would not see her niece alive again.

In the operating room, Dr. Newman opened Batchimeg's chest and was astounded at what she saw. She said, "This is a heart you just don't get to see. Amazing." She proceeded to fix what needed to be fixed, using creativity in the process due to the uniqueness of Batchimeg's heart. Surgical repairs were accomplished, left atrium trimmed down to size, and valve replaced; all amazing conquests of their own. For 12 long hours, Dr. Newman was brilliant, focused, and creative.

The moment of truth came as the doctor took her off the bypass machine, having her blood flow through her heart again. The Operating Room became silent. It was into the evening hours, yet everyone was as sharp as a pin, waiting for her heart to beat. And there it was! A heart beating on its own! But she had been on cardiac bypass for several hours, each hour adding to the possibility of bleeding around the heart.

After the initial cheers, the room once again became silent as all eyes were glued on Batchimeg's heart. The oozing of blood started, as we had all feared. Attempts at stopping the bleeding were unsuccessful, which meant putting Batchimeg back on the bypass machine while thinking about what to do next. Dr. Newman continued to do her thing until the heart was ready to come off bypass for the second time. Again, all eyes on Batchimeg's heart, first waiting for it to beat on its own, a sigh of relief rather than a celebration. This time the bleeding started a bit sooner and was a bit worse. Back on and off bypass, a third and final time. Initially, the doctors thought that coming off the bypass machine once would be too much.

REDIRECTING

Throughout the surgery, Dr. Newman and Greg Lammle, her husband of 28 years and her physician assistant, worked seamlessly as a team, as though able to read the others' mind. Now there was silence. Dr. Newman broke the silence by saying, "If we keep putting her back on bypass the bleeding will continue to get worse each time we take her off." Greg agreed. Dr. Newman continued, "Batchimeg will die if we put her back on and off bypass and she'll die if the bleeding continues and right now there is nothing we can do to stop the bleeding."

At this point, many surgeons would have quit, deciding that they had done what they could. After all, everyone knew it was going to be a risky surgery. But Dr. Newman's passion and calling kicked into high gear. Batchimeg was not just a patient, she was a person who Dr. Newman cared about. She said, "I have an idea. Let's use her own tissue to make a 'pocket' around her heart which will collect the blood. Then I'll put a flexible tube that will go from the pocket back into the heart. With time, the bleeding will stop. Until then, she will essentially be giving herself a constant transfusion of her own blood." How did she come up with that? Dr. Newman completed the task and when she was finished doing something she had never done before, she looked at Batchimeg's heart and said, "I hope I don't have to explain to anyone why this heart looks like it does!" No one cared what it looked like because it worked!

It was time to talk with the extended family in the waiting room. During the surgery, the family and friends had been given scant reports on what was happening. They had not heard a word for several hours. As I walked into the waiting room, one look at the tired faces, troubled eyes, disheveled hair and clothes, I saw a glimpse of their anguish. The longer the time lingered, the more assured they were that Batchimeg must not have made it through surgery. They were all anxious and fearful to see me. When I told them that Batchimeg had made it through surgery, their minds could not comprehend my words. Shortly thereafter, Dr. Newman came into the room with a wide smile on her face, saying that Batchimeg had survived surgery! It was only then that they were all able to trust their bodies and allow relief to seep through their pores. They could breathe. Hugs, tears, and smiles filled the room.

After I talked with the family and looked in on Batchimeg one last time in the Intensive Care Unit, I went to my parents' home and crashed in bed, knowing Batchimeg still had a very long night ahead of her before we could say she would recover. I returned in the morning, expecting to see Munkhbayar awake and Batchimeg on a ventilator. What I actually saw stopped me in my tracks and caused my heart to sink to my toes. The curtain around Batchimeg's bed was closed and her ventilator was outside of the curtains. God, this cannot be happening. After everything You brought Batchimeg through, why have her die now?

Suddenly the curtain was opened, and what I saw was mind-blowing! Miraculous even. My heart moved back up my chest as my jaw dropped to my knees. Batchimeg was sitting up in bed, drinking water! Dr. Rios was standing by her bedside and I moved to stand next to him as he told me, "We were very concerned throughout the night. She had a very stormy few hours." He and I were baffled at the quick turn-around. Then I remembered the prayer warriors, still at work in the church across the street from the hospital, not quite having finished their 24 hours of continuous prayer. As soon as Batchimeg saw me, she flashed me one of her smiles, and I knew I was one link in a chain, one piece of a puzzle that God was using to sculpt Batchimeg's life.

The power of one is evident in so many people who were a part of Batchimeg getting the care she needed to live. Dr. Kirk Milhoan and I meeting at a medical conference, Kirk performing screenings in Mongolia for heart defects, having an open slot to bring someone to Fargo, the father willing to do whatever was necessary to keep his daughter alive, the ticket agent who got Kevin and me on the plane in Beijing, the flight attendant who ultimately let us on the plane in Mongolia, Dr. Newman and her surgical team, Dr. Bob Brunsvold who wouldn't accept the CEO's decision to deny care to the Mongolians, the host church, host family, church coordinator, everyone involved in hospital care and rehabilitation, the prayer warriors, people donating money to cover travel costs, children with lemonade stands to raise money, Kevin covering the story that became front line news on more than one occasion and brought the entire Fargo-Moorhead community together for a common good. As Doc told PK in *The Power of One*, "Without the sun, the moon would be a dark circle, but with cooperation, moon light."

Once our patients had recovered, they were both able to go on outings and experience more than they could have imagined: fishing, canoeing, jet skiing, swimming. At a Concordia College (Cobbers) Corn Feed, they ate corn on the cob for the first time and were named honorary Cobbers. North Dakota Governor John Hoeven gave them certificates making them honorary citizens of North Dakota. While relaxing in a lounger in the backyard of LaMae's home, Batchimeg tearfully said, "We are hooked on people's love, taking care of us like their own children. You gave life back to me."

When it came time to start the two-day journey home to Mongolia, the airport was full of the people who had been most intimately involved. Most people, from children to grown men, were crying as hugs were freely given. Dr. Bob Brunsvold said, "This supports my faith. I've received more than I've given." As this was shortly before the 9/11 bombings, we were all able to be at the departure gate. When the final boarding call was made and all the other passengers had boarded, there was no more stalling. Munkhbayar was the last to board as he came out of the jet way three times to wave "one more time" to his new friends. Batchimeg and Munkhbayar came from Mongolia with no chance to live long in their country. Now they were returning home to start a new chapter in their lives.

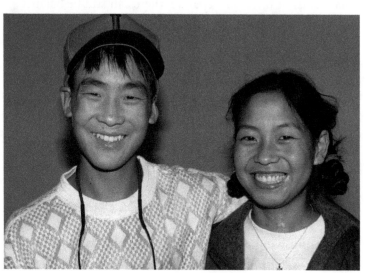

Dr. Roxanne Newman was one very large drop of water with her talent, ingenuity, and love for people. Roxanne exemplifies someone who lives her vocation, calling, and passion. Somehow, she is able to do this by keeping balance in her life. In a December 14, 2013, article in INFORUM, the online Fargo Forum entitled, "Women of Influence: Newman's Influence Extends to Individual Patients and Cardiovascular Field," written by Sherri Richards, Roxanne was asked what triggered her love of medicine at an early age when no one in her family was in the medical field. She replied, "How do you know what color you like?" I love her response! There are some things we just can't explain, questions with no answers. Roxanne has pioneered many areas of cardiothoracic surgery, including robotic surgery. In addition, she finds time to ride her horses, play viola in chamber orchestra at her church, learn bass, and fly a plane. She manages to live a balanced life. She acknowledges that she can't completely leave her work behind but, in her words, "It doesn't mean you can't have balance. Even if it's not separate, there can still be balance."

Recently, she told me that she calls the procedure done on Batchimeg, the "Batchimeg Baffle" and has used the procedure on other patients with aortic dissections and bleeding caused by poor clotting. She said, "I actually have had no mortalities on any patient that we needed to do the 'Batchimeg Baffle.' Who knew a sick little girl would impact so many of us." The continuing ripple effect of the power of one. Batchimeg was drenched in a waterfall.

Today, Batchimeg remains healthy and lives in Mongolia with her husband and two daughters. She calls Mongolia her home but says she is from Fargo, North Dakota.

CONCEPT 6

The power of one is transcended through the power of Jesus Christ. Without His power, how did one person start a chain of events in Mongolia that, within 10 years, changed the country from not being able to safely provide heart surgery, to one with a 95 percent survival with heart surgery? Without His power, how can one attempt to explain why Batchimeg is alive? The only way I can make sense of it is that the original power of one is Jesus Christ. Jesus can use all of us, whether we believe in Him or not. I don't know if the man at the ticket counter in China or the flight attendant in Mongolia are Christians. What I do know is that God used them, along with innumerable others, to ultimately change, in a positive way, thousands of lives.

REDIRECTING

Been close enough to feel the breeze
The coolness of the mist come over me
Heard the falling water
Like thunder through the trees

One step from unveiling
The glory of this mystery
Scared of plunging into the unknown

Where Your love comes pouring down
Like a waterfall
Capsizing my heart and soul
Your love comes pouring down
Life a waterfall
Baptizing . . .

You were the one drawing me
To move from my complacency
To let Your Spirit come cascading over me

Finally unveiling
The glory of this mystery
Plunging into the unknown
It's overwhelming

Where Your love comes pouring down
Like a waterfall

—Solomon's Wish, *Waterfall*

Conclusion

The Mission, the song by the Newsboys I noted earlier, started us on a path that has landed us here. Our mission today, as the Newsboys share, joins the mission of Christians from the time of Jesus' birth, indeed, "passing a baton forward through time," generation to generation, "lifting Your love higher." As the baton is being passed from one generation to the next, we each have our own torch that can be used to pass on the flame of our vocation, calling, and passion to those around us—to take over the work we can no longer do. The beauty of a torch is that by lighting someone else's, my flame is not extinguished. I can still use my flame, even though I will be moving in a different direction.

"The commission from God's lips to our ears," comes directly from Jesus, the initial flame, power of one, out-of-the-box thinker. When a Pharisee asked Jesus which commandment is the greatest, as we see in Matthew 22:37-40, Jesus responded, "'You shall love the Lord your God with all your heart and with all your soul, and with all your mind.' This is the greatest and first commandment. And a second is like it: 'You shall love your neighbor as yourself.'" Can it be that simple? When Jesus commissioned the disciples, He was basically starting the process of passing the baton to the people who would continue His work, passing a torch burning with love and passion.

Considered the Great Commission by many, Matthew 28:18-20 reminds us of Jesus' words: "All authority in heaven and on earth has been given to me. Go therefore and make disciples of all nations, baptizing them in the name of the Father and of the Son and of the Holy Spirit, and teaching them to obey everything that I have commanded you. And remember, I am with you always, to the end of the age." In a nutshell, Jesus was telling them to spread the word; love your Lord your God with everything you have in you, and love your neighbor as yourself. He doesn't stop there, however, as He says that He will always be with us, there is nowhere we can go to escape His Presence. Even if we don't know it, He's with us.

What ever happened to a passion I could live for?
What became of the flame that made me feel more?
And when did I forget that . . .

I was made to love You
I was made to find You
I was made just for You
Made to adore You
I was made to love and be loved by You
You were here before me

CONCLUSION

You were waiting on me
And You said You'd keep me,
never would You leave me
I was made to love
And be loved by You

—TobyMac, *Made to Love*

Knowing He is with us accomplishes many things, the most important of which is to offer us hope. There are times in life when we could feel hopeless; instead, I choose hope. In Urban Rescue's song, *Recreate*, three words resonate: "Hope illuminates tomorrow." Knowing there is hope in every circumstance makes it easier to step out into the unknown, risking the comfortable, trying something new. I am trying to find my way to the point where I expect difficulties—that part is easy for me—and when they come, to not let them alter my course of walking with God, feeling His presence every step of the way (that's the hard part).

When everything else is stripped away, Christ is still there for us. God does not promise us a life without difficulties; He does promise to be with us through it all even if He may seem far away at the time. Hope allows us to see beyond the crisis of the present moment, knowing that God is in charge of the big picture. No matter what happens in this life, we know that God has promised us a better future. He sealed that promise with the birth and subsequent death and resurrection of His very own Son. However, we are not meant to sit around, waiting for a better future. We are all a masterpiece, crafted by God's own hands, created to bring hope and love to all in our own unique way. In Romans 5:1-5 we read, "Therefore, since we are justified by faith, we have peace with God through our Lord Jesus Christ, through whom we have obtained access to this grace in which we stand; and we boast in our hope of sharing the glory of God. And not only that, but we also boast in our sufferings, knowing that suffering produces endurance, and endurance produces character, and character produces hope, and hope does not disappoint us, because God's love has been poured into our hearts through the Holy Spirit that has been given to us."

As I walk this great unknown
Questions come and questions go
Was there purpose for the pain
Did I cry these tears in vain
I don't wanna live in fear
I wanna trust that You are near
Trust Your grace can be seen
In both triumph and tragedy

I have this hope
In the depth of my soul
In the flood or the fire
You are with me and You won't let go

—Tenth Avenue North, *I Have This Hope*

There is a particular incident in my life that solidified my belief that there is always hope. Less than four months after my Traumatic Brain Injury, I was at a Mount Carmel

Ministries (MCM) family week with my parents and brother. At this point in time, my short-term memory was shorter than a pancake, and my word-finding ability was significantly affected, making it impossible to speak a complete sentence fluently. When people looked in my eyes, they did not see my usual sparkle. In its place was the look of someone who was not present in the moment.

MCM is like the vast majority of camps in Minnesota—on a lake. I was watching a soccer game when I heard a desperate plea coming from the beach. "Medical emergency! We need help!" Without thinking, I ran to the beach and found people surrounding a man who was in shock, not responding to anyone. My traumatized brain switched the direction of neurons to flow toward the medical knowledge section, which jumped into action. I took the lead, directing others, with complete fluency.

Someone said, "He was on the back of a Jet Ski, facing backwards to spot for tubers. The rope from the Jet Ski to the tube was wrapped around his leg. The driver did not know when he took off at full speed. The rope tightened around his leg, throwing him into the water! We pulled him to shore but he hasn't responded to us!" A nurse had arrived shortly before me and ordered someone to get a medical kit.

I looked at the pale man, asked for his name, and said, "Joel, you're going to be fine. I'm a doctor." I explained what happened and when I said that there was bruising from rope burn, he slowly opened his eyes and said, "My leg is still attached? I thought it was ripped off."

"No," was my reply, "you're going to have quite a bruise, but your leg is still securely attached to your body." He flashed a slight smile while everyone around took a deep breath as faces etched with concern turned to smiles. At the same time, the medical kit arrived and I took his vital signs.

When I told him his blood pressure, his smile widened as he said, "Now I really know I'm in good hands. That's exactly what it was last week when I went to the doctor!" The ambulance arrived, Joel was loaded into the back as I gave my report to the emergency responders, the doors were closed, and the ambulance drove away.

As I looked around, all eyes were focused on me. At that moment, I did not understand what had just happened. For the first time since the accident, my speech was fluent, the sparkle in my eyes was back, and I had just performed the duties of a physician. However, when I looked back at the crowd, including my family, as the ambulance drove away, the sparkle disappeared and I could no longer put words together to make a sentence. What had happened? From a medical standpoint, I can say that I went into medical mode, tapped into a part of my brain that had not been affected by the accident, and did what I was trained to do. From a spiritual standpoint, I believe God was giving me hope. And I will hold onto hope for the rest of my life. It took me a couple of days to understand what happened as people filled me in on the details.

Joel came back to camp later that night. When he was evaluated in the Emergency Room, the doctor said, "Whoever took care of you on the beach did everything necessary.

CONCLUSION

There's nothing more we need to do except give you some pain medicine." At the end of the camp week, Joel gave me a card, expressing his thanks. Upon receiving his card, it sunk in—my medical knowledge is fine, and there is hope that someday I will be able to return to my vocation, calling, and passion.

Hearing God's plan for us is not a one-time event, but rather a daily discipline. Often, to be able to listen, we need to be still. Psalm 46:10, "Be still, and know that I am God!" In this context, the Hebrew meaning of "be still" is to stop striving, let go, and surrender. Sometimes we think if we aren't doing something, we're wasting time. Quite the opposite! We're commanded to take time to stop doing and be still. Think of the freedom that gives us!

Open Hands by Urban Rescue is the song I chose to end the book with as we move forward into the world, living a life of significance with passion and a sense of calling. Recently, a close friend said that sometimes we hold our fists tight, not letting go of what we think we need to hang onto and not accepting what we really need. Oh, my goodness. That is me more often than I would like to admit. Opening our fists is usually not a quick, one-time event. As we gradually open our hands, we let go of what is holding us down and we let in what will set us free to live the life we were born to live, with nothing left to prove! I am a work in progress and wish I could say that I am a great example of everything I write. We are on this trek together.

I hope within the pages of this book you have been remind-ed that you are loved, unique with a calling, empowered to follow your passion, and that within you lies the power of one. I also hope *you* will be motivated and encouraged to get involved in the world in a positive way—whether across the street or across the ocean. There will be roadblocks along our journey, but they don't have to stop us—instead, they can be used to change our direction. It can be frightening stepping out of our comfort zone, stepping into the Jordan River, leaving behind a job and following our vocation—indeed, daring to think outside the box. Sometimes it's hard to balance our responsibilities with our calling and passion, but I believe it's doable when we take the time to look deeply into our lives and decide how we want to be remembered when we're gone. We can be a drop of water that starts a waterfall, or join a waterfall that is already raging. Ultimately, when we listen to what our lives are telling us and where God is leading us, every journey we begin has the possibility of bringing us to where our deep gladness meets the world's deep hunger.

CONCLUSION

I'll never catch Your light
Living with knuckles white
Keeping my fist held tight
I'll never touch Your heart
Or take in all You are
Trying to hide my scars
I'm letting go of holding on

Here I am with open hands
I have nothing left to prove
God, I give it all to you
Empty me of everything
Till there's nothing left but You
I just want to live for You
With open hands

I'm finally giving up
I'm placing all my trust
Into a higher love
You're dreaming bigger dreams
You have a plan for me
And though I cannot see

My hands for Your glory, my hands for Your glory
Lifted high, lifted high to You
My life for Your glory, my life for Your glory
All of me, All of me for You

—Urban Rescue, *Open Hands*

Questions to Consider When You Are Being Redirected:

1. Who am I?

2. What am I doing here?[8]

3. What signs or messages do I hear from God or others who might be helping to direct my path?

4. Do I have an open mind and heart when it comes to the possibility of being redirected?

5. How will my life be impacted if I follow this new course, or if I reject it?

6. Who in my life can offer honest feedback about the possibilities that lie in my future?

Endnotes

[1]L'Engle, Madeleine (1962), *A Wrinkle in Time.* New York, NY: Dell Publishing Co., Inc.

[2]Buechner, Frederick (1973). *Wishful Thinking: A Theological ABC.* Harper & Row.

[3]Palmer, Parker J. (2000). *Let Your Life Speak: Listening for the Voice of Vocation.* San Francisco, CA: Jossey-Bass.

[4]Young, Sarah (2004). *Jesus Calling: Enjoying Peace in His Presence.* Nashville, Tennessee: Thomas Nelson, Inc.

[5]Palmer, Parker (2000). *Let Your Life Speak: Listening for the Voice of Vocation.* San Francisco, CA: Jossey-Bass.

[6]Zaentz, Saul (Producer), & Babenco, Hector (Director). (1991). *At Play in the Fields of the Lord* [Motion picture]. United States: Universal Home Video.

[7]Milchan, Arnon (Producer), & Avildsen, John G. (Director). (1992). *The Power of One* [Motion picture]. United States: Warner Brothers.

[8]Hoppock, Amy (2017). *32 Questions,* Boise, ID: Aloha Publishing.

Acknowledgments

In addition to all those who have shaped my life and are part of my stories, there are so many people to thank for their role in making my book a reality. It is impossible to name everyone for whom I am grateful as that would double the size of the book.

To my family, there are not enough words to thank you. Mom and Dad (Dale & Lu Vitalis), you have watched over me, prayed for me, loved me, challenged me, and on rare occasion, reprimanded me! I love you, need you, and am proud to be your daughter. My sister, Kathy Hoffman, you are my best friend and have been a role model since we were youngsters. Being an introvert, I was able to ride on your extrovert coattails. This book would not be what it is without your editing help. My brother-in-law, Mark Hoffman, thanks for being a great husband to Kathy and fathering two wonderful girls, in addition to making great homemade pizza! Sarah, we bonded at your birth in a unique way that I so treasure. I am so proud of how you have grown through difficult situations that life has thrown your way. Our common love of sports will persist, even though I can no longer participate. ATI. Amy, I was out of the country when you were born, but I think we have made up time for that lost first week of your life. Your optimism, compassion, and humor fill a room. I treasure the bond we have in a common desire to help the "least of these," outcasts, those who need a hand to help pull them up and empower them to live a full life. MUL. My sister, Beth Vitalis, my dear sister, we have shared a lot of ups and downs together and have come out the other end stronger. Who would have thought that our mutual love of sciences and medicine would bring us together in Kenya! I love our carefree times together and that you accept me for who I am, flaws and all. Thank you for honoring me with the role of crew chief for your 100-mile runs. My brother-in-law, Joe McDonald, thanks for being a great husband to Beth. Keep making the best homemade pie in the world! Steven Vitalis, my dear brother, you have taught me so much about life. You have persevered with dignity and grace through the difficulties of living with autism, in a world not always willing to think outside the box. You are a shining example of how someone with autism can make a change in the world. And, thanks to all my cousins and their families who have supported me in various ways when most needed. Ashki, my constant furry companion, thank you for loving me unconditionally like only a dog can do.

To Aloha Publishing: Maryanna Young, Jennifer Regner, and Anna McHargue; you have graciously given your time and energy to help see me through this project. Maryanna, your love and integrity show that there really are angels on earth. Anna, editor extraordinaire, you have moved your job into

ACKNOWLEDGMENTS

your vocation. Anna, without you, I would not believe that I truly am an author. Your editing skills, encouragement, and gentleness have made this book more than I could ever imagine or do on my own. You are an amazing editor and an amazing person. I am so proud and humbled (is that an oxymoron?) to have the opportunity to be on a team with you. Knowing you're a 49ers fan when you picked me up from the airport wearing a Vikings shirt, I knew I had lifelong friend. You will always be the special sauce to this sesame seed.

To my Aloha Dream Team, you have helped me see myself more clearly than ever before. Maryanna Young, Amy Hoppock, and Dave Weitz, you have been my rock, my sanity, my reality, making me face my demons, and bringing in humor when needed. And emojis. And dance. And tears when they were most needed. Because of your help, I am personally at a better place than I have been for decades. And the grace and wonder of it all is that even though you know everything about me, you still love me. LYM

To the Maui team that started the book process, without our time in Maui and all the God-ordained events that occurred, this book would not exist. Judy Siegle, my friend, thank you for inviting me to travel with you to Maui. Thank you for the support you have given me in so many ways that have allowed me to follow my calling and write this book. Thanks for sticking with me all these decades. Maryanna Young, thank you for inviting me to Boise, Idaho, and then insisting I follow through. You are the catalyst for the book's existence. Kim Fletcher, thank you for all the wisdom you passed along about writing a book and encouraging me to set a lunch date with Kirk and Kim Milhoan. Where do I even start with Drs. Kirk and Kim Milhoan! Reconnecting with you in Maui and sharing mutual past pains that were beyond our control was one of the most healing times in my life. Kirk, seeing you preach and teach the Bible in a poverty-stricken area of Maui was inspiring. The combination of the entire Maui contingent was the perfect storm for me to pursue writing this book. To have this experience come full circle, back to Maui, is such a blessing. Speaking at Calvary Chapel South Maui's Women's Retreat recently was life changing. A huge thanks to Tayla, Brandy, Amy, Kim, Judy, and Roxanne for ignoring the "Keep Out" sign, trekking across narrow bridges and tough terrain so I could live my dream of swimming under a waterfall!

Christian songs with great lyrics have played a huge role in keeping me from falling off the ledge. To all Christian musicians, I thank you for following your calling, which fans many flames through your lyrics. Shane and Shane, thank you for starting my new vocation of being a road doctor for Christian musicians. Shane and Kellie, Shane and Beth, I am blessed to be your friend. To Jeremy Camp and band members Toby Friesen and Leif Skartland, thanks for finding a drum set for me! Thanks to the musicians who have allowed me a small peek into your world; Phil and Mallory Wickham, Mat Kearney, Sara Groves, Bebo Norman, Matt Maher, Rend Collective, Urban Rescue, Mike and Lisa Gungor, Dave Lubbin, Elizabeth Hunnicutt, and Amy Howson. To Matt Best and Echo Ministries, thanks for all you do to bring Christian concerts to lesser-known venues. I would also like to thank Jon Foreman of Switchfoot, who allowed my cousin Wade and me to catch him as he stepped off the balcony at First Ave. in Minneapolis.

ACKNOWLEDGMENTS

For those who have been involved in my health care, bringing me to a better place, I thank you. Dawn Stover, Dr. Alex Mendez, Dr. Robert Olson, Dr. Paula Bergloff, Lorene Peterson, Janet Grove, and Nan Kennelly. You are awesome!

Thank you to all the people who read and reviewed the first portion of my book in advance of publication. Your feedback encouraged me to keep writing.

To all the people who have worked alongside me in the trenches, helping the least of these, thank you. There are too many to name them all. Thanks to Dr. Dave and Jody Stevens, Dr. Dan and Cindy Tolan, Dr. Bob and Dora Wesche, Dr. Michael and Kay Johnson, Dr. Marty and Ann Graber, Robyn Moore, Susan Carter, Wendy Webb, Diane Terpstra, Faith Shingledecker, Joy Phillips, Dr. Tina Slusher, Kia Channer, Jim and Grace Harrelson, Dr. Paul and Jan Jones, Karen O'Neill, Tana Koch, Dr. Michael VanRooyen, Mindy Coatney, Noelle Tope Merritt, Christy Rich, Global Health Ministries, and Mount Carmel Ministries. And the family who started with me from the beginning, Roger and Joan Lindholm, Leah, Jamie, Ellie, and Ana.

To the teachers and schools who have helped shape me throughout the years, a huge thank you: Oak Grove Lutheran School, Concordia College, Johns Hopkins School of Medicine, Methodist Hospital Residency program; Marc Langseth, Paul Budd, Marilyn Nielsen, Arvid Berg, Robin Altenbernd, the late Elinor Torstveit, Ivan Johnson, Patty and Shannon Jung, Dr. Vern Tolo, Dr. Jean Kan, the late Dr. Henry Seidel, Dr. Kim Bateman, the late Dr. Dick Bick, the late Dr. Tony Spagnolo, and Dr. Craig Christianson.

REDIRECTING

To my fellow Residents, it was wonderful sharing our lives for three years. Dr. Roger and Joan Lindholm, Dr. Doug and Anne Smith, Dr. Phil and Eileen Disraeli, Dr. Brian Prokosch, Dr. Jeremy and Nancy Springer. Jeremy, I still owe you a night of call.

To Nidaros Lutheran Church, thank you for being my community of faith, inviting me in as family. I love you all!

Thank you to my friends who have been with me throughout my journey, the families of Lochers, Ruehles, Zenders, and Adams.

Roxanne and Curt Thompson, Sara and Pat Kalk, Dan Ruhland, Matt Carlson, Carmen Keller, Dr. Mary Jane Tetzloff, Dr. Alison LaFrence, Dr. Lucinda (Cindy) Bateman, Karoline Pierson, Judy Siegle, Peggy Isakson, John and Heidi Parkes, Cindy and Dave Meldahl, Lynn Hunstad, Beth Dahlberg Luby, Joslin Forness Bullock, Janet Black Rogne, Carrie Bowman, Nancy Bick, Heide Apedaile, Kurt Nelson and all the Happy Hearts, Allyson Greene and the rest of my East Rosebud friends. A special thank you to Lois Dalthorp and her family for the use of their Montana cabin as a getaway to write and recharge.

A special note of thanks to Kevin Wallevand. You are a drop of water that has started many waterfalls, and I am blessed to have been able to drop in on some. Thanks for your friendship through-out the years.

Above all, I give all the glory to God; Father, Son, and Holy Spirit. Despite my sins, Your love never fails me, and Your presence always surrounds me.

SUSAN MARY VITALIS, M.D.

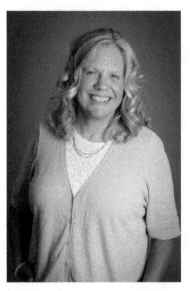

Dr. Susan Vitalis has a passion for helping the helpless, bringing hope to the hopeless, and empowering those who feel powerless. After graduating from Concordia College in Moorhead, Minnesota, and Johns Hopkins School of Medicine in Baltimore, Maryland, she completed a Family Medicine residency in Minneapolis, Minnesota. Dr. Vitalis subsequently split her time between Minnesota and other parts of the world, including Kenya, Somalia, Southern Sudan, Rwanda, Central African Republic, Bosnia-Herzegovina, Kosovo, Albania, Mongolia, and Tibet. In addition to her international work, Dr. Vitalis has volunteered locally in numerous capacities. Throughout her life, Dr. Vitalis has been faced with many unforeseen events and obstacles that continually change the path of her vocation, calling, and passion. With each stumbling block, she has ultimately found her way to a place of feeling God's presence and love while listening to Him whisper her name, giving reassurance that He has a plan.

For more about Dr. Vitalis' work in Southern Sudan, read "Bullets, Bats, and a Bomb Shelter" inside the book *Don't Miss Your Boat: Living Your Life with Purpose in the Real World*, by Maryanna Young and Kim Fletcher.

CPSIA information can be obtained
at www.ICGtesting.com
Printed in the USA
LVHW04s2236230418
574630LV00024B/379/P

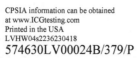

9 780999 760208